M.E.

How to Live with It

DR ANNE MACINTYRE

Thorsons
An Imprint of HarperCollins*Publishers*

Thorsons
An Imprint of HarperCollins*Publishers*
77–85 Fulham Palace Road,
Hammersmith, London W6 8JB

First published by Unwin Hyman 1988
This edition published 1992
1   3   5   7   9   10   8   6   4   2

A catalogue record for this book
is available from the British Library

ISBN 0 7225 2624 5

Typeset by Harper Phototypesetters Limited
Northampton, England
Printed in Great Britain by
HarperCollinsManufacturing Glasgow

Contents

Foreword

To have ME is to experience hell twice over, firstly through the devastation of the disease itself, and secondly through the lack of diagnosis, information and support that most sufferers are still having to endure.

In the early days of my illness I dragged myself to the local library and combed the medical reference books for some indication of the name and possible causes of this ghastly affliction. I found nothing. My doctor and the various specialists I saw were hardly more helpful. I was eventually told it was a 'virus' – a vague-sounding diagnosis if ever there was one – and that was it. I was given no advice excepting 'total rest', and was offered none of the support which I so desperately needed. On the contrary, I, like so many sufferers before me, was made to feel guilty for my illness, as if I had brought it upon myself. The horrific mental symptoms were put down to reactive depression: had I had an upset recently? An unhappy love affair perhaps? As a single parent, wasn't life a bit much for me? The fact that, until my illness, my life had never been happier or more fulfilled was overlooked. My real mistake, of course, was to have developed an illness which cannot be diagnosed by simple blood tests, which has a bewildering array of strange and sometimes vague symptoms, and for which there is no magic cure.

By the time I had completed the first round of doctors my isolation was almost complete. Not surprisingly, family and friends found it difficult to understand a disease which had no name, no visible symptoms, makes you come apart mentally, yet often leaves you looking perfectly well. Rather than test their loyalty beyond reasonable bounds, I pretended my illness wasn't happening. I covered up the gaping holes in my life with lies and evasions: while I slept all day my answering machine said I was out; when I stumbled over words or walked into things I joked about having had a late night; and my social life was reduced to almost nothing by constantly pleading a previous engagement.

I began to live the life of a recluse – a lonely, isolated and desperate recluse. Looking back, it was a living nightmare. Yet many sufferers have experienced far, far worse: alienation, denigration, loss of employment and the break-up of relationships.

It is my ambition and that of my colleagues in the ME Action Campaign that ME sufferers should never again have to endure their illness in such appalling isolation and ignorance. Although much progress has been made in the recognition of the disease, there is still a very long way to go. In particular, there is an urgent need to reach the many sufferers who, though desperate for inform-ation and support, still do not know where to turn.

This book should do much to help those people. It provides the widest and most detailed information on ME yet published. Anne Macintyre, who is both a doctor and a sufferer, has explained the disease in the light of the latest available research, and taken an impartial look at all the various therapies and treatments currently in use.

I hope this book will prevent sufferers from making the mistakes that I and so many other desperate people have made. I wasted much energy, not to mention money, on traipsing up and down Harley Street seeing numerous doctors, both orthodox and alternative, who swore they knew exactly what was wrong with me (their diagnoses nearly always differed), who pressed me into following their ineffective, bizarre, even dangerous remedies, and who, in the end, left me worse off both physically and financially.

None of the treatments and therapies discussed in this book will effect a miracle cure, for none exists, but all have been tried by ME sufferers and in some cases, though inevitably not all, provided improvement or relief. All of us who have battled with ME over any length of time know the importance of approaching the disease from many different angles simultaneously – diet, supplementation, and lifestyle – and of experimenting to find out what suits us as individuals. This book provides the information on which to build a programme to suit yourself and your unique set of difficulties and problems. Self-help, as most ME sufferers learn through long and hard experience, is the only way forward.

It is unfortunate that sufferers of such a debilitating disease should be thrown back on their own resources, and yet, since self-help is by far the best way of tackling the illness, it is no bad thing. We expect too much of medicine and science. Indeed, we are the victims as well as the beneficiaries of this scientific age. We find ourselves in a situation where, if routine tests cannot pick up an illness, it cannot exist. Textbooks are consulted as if they were written in stone. The medical profession feels bound to give answers even where there are none.

Yet leading scientists will always be the first to admit that what is known is always exceeded by what is unknown. It is sometimes forgotten that the intricacies of the immune system are only now beginning to be unravelled. And in the field of enteroviruses, which are heavily implicated in ME, virtually all work ceased after the development of the polio vaccine in 1954. Research does not continue in a smooth curve, but in fits and starts instigated by necessity.

Other diseases have had to battle for recognition – notably multiple sclerosis, an illness which also responds to self-help. And other diseases have been misunderstood – isolated cases of polio were often labelled neurotic or hysteric in origin. All became accepted in time.

But however slow acceptance may be in coming, there is the consolation that the majority of ME sufferers do eventually recover. This may offer small comfort to those in the thick of the illness who can see nothing but months of gloom ahead, and for those who have already endured years of unremitting symptoms, but the facts do point to eventual improvement for most.

I have had enormous ups and downs, but experimentation with many of the treatments and remedies described here has brought slow improvement and ever-quicker recovery from relapse. Furthermore, the more I have learnt about the illness, the more I have been able to come to grips with it.

I hope that, for all the sufferers who read this book, it brings a glimmer of light to the end of the tunnel.

Clare Francis

Preface to the 1992 Edition

In the three years since I finished work for the first edition of this book, there have appeared many new medical papers about M.E., more often called Chronic Fatigue Syndrome (CFS) in Britain now. There has been a lot of writing from physicians and psychiatrists, who hypothesize that the illness is due to depression, or overbreathing, or deconditioning from too much rest. On the other side, very valuable objective medical research is being done, early results of which are confirming that M.E. is an organic disease, with demonstrable pathology in muscle and brain. But still the arguments rage – is M.E. caused by untreated depression, with a virus as an opportunist? Or is it a persistent viral infection in genetically susceptible people, with depression as a major secondary effect?

With the increasing use of 'chronic fatigue' as a description of the illness, I believe that there is now confusion between

1. Myalgic Encephalomyelitis, the condition described in many past outbreaks, carefully described by Dr Melvin Ramsay, probably caused by a relative of polio virus, and
2. Chronic Fatigue Syndrome, which encompasses many fatigue states (some of which may be depression in disguise), some post-viral fatigue syndromes, some chronic overbreathing syndromes, and some myalgic encephalomyelitis.

Research projects are currently underway, whose final results will not appear in print before this book goes to press. By the time this book is published I hope that further important studies on the abnormalities in the brain, in particular the hypothalamus and its connections, will have been published.

I address this book mainly to sufferers from M.E., but hope that it will be helpful to anyone with any post-viral fatigue state or any chronic fatigue syndromes. If the information on research is difficult to understand, I apologize; I have found the task of compiling it, and translating 'medicalese' into plain English, a great strain on my brain, and a good test of cognitive non-function!

I would like to thank all those who have supplied useful information, and acknowledge the help from IFMEA (International Federation of M.E. Associations).

Anne Macintyre
March 1992

Preface to the 1988 Edition

There may be 100,000 people in Britain today, who are suffering from a strange illness which nobody yet understands. This illness can have a devastating effect on one's life.

My own story is a typical example: Five years ago I was able to work full-time in a busy hospital department, and to spend my free time gardening, decorating my home, socializing, and generally living a full life. I went to Scotland every year, and was able to achieve a whole day's hill-walking, maybe 18 miles. Like most people, I got colds in winter, and sometimes felt worn out after a busy day.

Four years ago, during a spell of very hard work while in India, I had a severe throat infection, but had to carry on working. After I returned home I remained unwell and tired for many weeks. Over the following three years I had periods of severe exhaustion alternating with short spells of nearly normal energy. My doctor could find nothing wrong, and did lots of tests, the results of which were all normal.

I had bouts of unexplained depression and feelings of utter 'awfulness', when I felt more ill than at any previous time in my life. I had to cut down my work to part-time, and to rest when not working. In the past I had found that a long walk in the countryside, or a swim, would lift me out of 'the blues'. But now any exercise was having a disastrous effect, and I had more benefit from spending the weekend just sitting in a chair. I knew that something was wrong, but no one could identify it. I feared that I was very neurotic, or maybe losing my mind.

Then a flu-like illness in August 1987, which featured fever and terrible muscle pains, seemed to plunge me into a worse state. Over the following three months I became unable to walk 50 yards without collapsing, my brain turned into cotton wool, I was unable to read or bear the sound of music; weird symptoms plagued me, including waking in the night with palpitations and loud noises in my head, my vision was often blurred, and I smelled things that were not there. But the overriding problem was the extreme exhaustion brought on by the simplest task, even brushing my hair, or chopping some vegetables.

But I am luckier than many sufferers. I found out in October 1987 from a physician that I had Myalgic Encephalomyelitis, and that it had probably started four years before, the bout in August being a severe relapse. I now knew where I stood, and was able to reorganize my life to try to cope with it. My condition improved a little, now that I could stop worrying about what was wrong. I still have to be very careful not to do too much, not to work in the garden or to try and walk far, even on a lovely day. I have not sold my mountain boots, though: I hope to use them again one day!

This disease has been described all over the world, principally in developed countries. In Britain it was known as Royal Free Disease (following an outbreak in the London hospital of that name in 1955) and also as Iceland Disease (where there was an outbreak in 1948–9). A rough estimate of the incidence at present is about 1 in 1,000 people. This makes it as prevalent as Parkinson's disease, and more common than Multiple Sclerosis. In countries where it does not appear to exist, this is because it is not yet recognized by the medical profession, and sufferers are given other labels. In Britain, Canada, Australia and New Zealand, the illness is known as Myalgic Encephalomyelitis; in the United States as Chronic Fatigue Syndrome. In this book I shall refer to it as M.E. or CFS.

I decided to write this book to provide useful information for people who think they may have M.E. and want to find out; for those who have been told they are suffering from it, but that there is no treatment; for friends and relations of sufferers; and for any doctors who still do not believe that M.E. is a genuine disease.

Many sufferers cannot obtain any diagnosis from their doctors, and even worse, some are labelled neurotic or hysterical after doing the rounds of various specialists. It is a sad fact of twentieth-century medicine that a diagnosis of disease depends more on laboratory tests and X-rays than on careful history-taking and examination. M.E. is a diagnosis based on the history of the patient's illness, and to date there is no single diagnostic test which gives a 100 per cent accurate answer.

The only branch of medicine that does not depend on tests or abnormal physical findings is psychiatry, and it is into this pigeon-hole that many M.E. patients are put. I wonder how many people are languishing in mental institutions who would be relieved to be told that they have a recognized organic disease, and whose health could improve from a regime that does not consist only of psychotropic drugs? This does not deny that very many people with M.E. do have mental symptoms as part of their disease, however.

Getting a diagnosis is one thing, and what a relief it is to know what is wrong with you. The next problem is: where do you get advice? Is there any cure? Is there anything that you can do for yourself to improve things? The answer to this last question is *yes*, and people with M.E. will cope a lot better if they stop expecting medical science to provide a cure, and instead set about organizing their own plan of action – or rather their plan of *in-action*; recovery from M.E. requires much less activity and more rest. One needs to learn to give *more* time to simply *being*, and *less* to *doing*.

If you who start to read this book have M.E., then the

chances are that you find it hard to concentrate for long.
If you decide that you have read enough for today, please
remember just two things:

1. You can certainly improve and have a good chance of
   some recovery.
2. The more you rest now and stop trying to achieve
   anything, the less frustrated you will be by your
   limitations, and the better your chances of improving.

We live in a culture which worships achievement and all
that goes with it. I can offer no proof nor scientific
explanation that M.E. is a disease of the twentieth
century and of 'developed' nations. But since the illness
is made worse by both physical and mental effort, I
wonder how prevalent it is in communities that practise
meditation, prayer and tranquility; such as in a Buddhist
monastery?

There is no doubt that M.E. follows on from a viral
infection in most sufferers, whether the infection is
noticed or not. But surely there must be other factors
involved? For why, in a family or group who all contract
a virus, does only one person go on to develop M.E.? At
the time of writing, there is no answer to this.

I see no reason for people who have this illness to wait
until it has been explained fully before having some
information and ideas about self-help.

This book brings together everything that is known so
far about M.E., and all known ways of coping with it.
Some methods are based on my own experience, others
I have gleaned from other sufferers. There is nothing
offered in the way of self-management that is harmful,
even though some methods have not yet been proven by
controlled medical trials. One problem in testing
treatments for M.E. is the up-and-down course of the
illness, which makes any improvement difficult to
evaluate. But we cannot wait forever for permission to try
and get better ourselves.

The Chinese have used acupuncture for thousands of

years, because they observed that it worked. They have not been troubled by the fact that no one has discovered exactly *how* it works; therefore if something seems to be helpful for a person with M.E. it is sensible to pass on the information to others. What is beneficial to one sufferer may not help another. However, *rest* is universally essential. Each person should learn to listen to his or her own body and co-operate with it to help recovery.

I hope that this book will be helpful for sufferers with M.E., and those who care for them. I hope it can give encouragement to anyone who has been compelled by this illness to come to a halt in a busy life, and who may be baffled and depressed by the experience. I have written from the viewpoint of a sufferer, and also as a doctor.

In recent years there has been a lot of valuable research into M.E.; the threads of understanding are starting to be woven together to make a picture of the disease process. More research projects are being planned, and several treatments are going to be tested in the USA. We can look forward to a time when the mystery of this devastating illness is solved, and hope that some definitive cure will become available.

Anne Macintyre
September 1988

Chapter 1

What is M.E.?

There are various names for this disease which causes profound exhaustion, pain, and mental confusion, and which leaves so much disability and suffering.

These are some of the names used:

Yuppie Flu – because it is mistakenly thought to affect mainly people who are high achievers
Chronic Epstein Barr Virus – in USA – used less commonly now
Chronic Fatigue Syndrome – CFS
Chronic Fatigue and Immune Dysfunction Syndrome – CFIDS
Icelandic Disease – from an outbreak in Iceland
Tapanui Flu – from an outbreak in New Zealand
Epidemic Neuromyesthenia
Royal Free Disease – from a 1955 London epidemic
Myalgic Encephalomyelitis

Whatever it is called, it is a very unpleasant condition. The main symptom is of *profound fatigue*, mental and physical, *made worse by exercise*, in combination with a variety of more bizarre symptoms, in a person who may look well, and in whom there are usually no abnormal signs on examination.

The effects of this disease can be devastating to someone who was previously active and led a full life. Not only are jobs lost and early retirement is necessary for many, but marriages may founder, relationships and friends be lost, and many hobbies and interests dropped. Even the most basic tasks of daily living may require such herculean effort that the patient cannot survive without help. Some M.E. people are prisoners in their bodies, and so the condition has been referred to by some as 'A living death'.

Added to all this suffering is the fact that for decades the disease was not recognized by the medical profession, apart from a few perceptive doctors, and patients were labelled as malingerers, neurotic, or mad.

Not surprisingly, a few who suffered from this condition have taken their own lives. They were not only very ill, but were denied the basic recognition of their illness and proper medical support.

Here is a fairly typical case history of M.E.:

Jean's Story

Jean is a dentist, married with two teenage sons. She was 41 when she had a bout of diarrhoea following a meal out at a hotel . . .

'I didn't seem to recover from that, I felt very weak. I was very overworked, looking after sick and elderly grandparents. This was about five years ago. I'd had a hysterectomy a year previously, which was followed by various complications, and I'd had a very nasty bout of flu just before the operation.

'After the diarrhoeal illness, my energy levels went down and up, and I would get attacks of ''flu'', low-grade fever, with tremendous exhaustion and weakness, lasting for several days.

'It was over a year before I was sent to hospital for tests. During this time my main symptoms were complete and utter exhaustion, severe aching muscle pains, inability to concentrate, inability to function normally – I was trying to run a job and a family. My ears became very irritated and sensitive to sound. I got very depressed, and iller and iller, and was more or less bedridden for about two years. I could just about get out to the shops and back, then collapsed in bed. I had to give up my job.

'I developed allergies to various foods which had not upset me previously. After becoming more and more ill for over a year following the diarrhoea illness, my GP referred me to an infectious diseases unit for tests. I had various blood tests, and the consultant thought I'd had a Coxsackie virus. He heard my story and told me I was ill with Myalgic Encephalomyelitis, and that he did not know how to make me better. I was too ill at the time to take much in, but at least, knowing I was ill, I could rest.

'The rest has been the main cure. For over two years I was so weak that all I could do was get out of bed and collect the things to prepare a meal and take them back to bed. I found cutting a carrot hard work. If I put coal on the fire it took so much energy I had to go back to bed again. I had great difficulty sleeping, because of the pain. I had two admissions to a psychiatric unit because of severe depression. Sometimes I was so tired that it was an effort to breathe. Once when I felt very ill my temperature went very low for a few weeks.

'It was about a year after I got a diagnosis before I started to get better. My improvement has not been steady – the relapses always occur after physical effort. Once, when I was a bit better, I had to stand in queues at a hospital clinic with a grandmother whom I was accompanying, then foolishly had to push the car, which wouldn't start, to take her home. I thought, with the adrenaline of the moment, that I could do it! I came home, collapsed into bed, and could not get up for a month. My brain packed in, I couldn't function, and it took me months to get over it.

'Last year I began to get a bit better. My GP thought that a little physiotherapy would do me good because I was so weak. It was disastrous, even hydrotherapy, although I felt great for the first week, but after 10 days the aching and slight fever came back.

'When I was very ill I had dreadful ulcers in my mouth, and Fungilin lozenges helped enormously. It was thought to be a Candida infection.

'I am now on a total ''no exercise'' campaign. As long as I lie or sit, I can function mentally. Even when I was at my worst, I tried to put clothes on every day, this kept my circulation going, and provided enough exercise to stop me seizing up.

'I found that complete bed rest when my temperature was up was beneficial, but only for a short time; when my temperature had settled I tried to get dressed every day.

'The first year of the illness I kept fighting it, so of course I just got worse. To begin with it was physical exhaustion. In the second year, I found the mental problems got worse. I couldn't finish a sentence I had started, and my brain switched off. It was so frustrating, I just wept. I felt completely useless, I was just a burden to everybody. I used to say to the boys ''put me out for the dustmen in a black plastic bag!'' '

Jean is now in the eighth year of the illness, but is slowly and steadily getting better. She works one half-day a week, and is able to go out some evenings with her family. Her food allergies have improved, but she finds that sticking to a wholefood diet with plenty of salads, not a lot of meat, and no bread, sugar or cakes, helps her. A large meat meal robs her of energy.

Her husband and children were very supportive. 'He got me better through the emotional side of it. When you are very ill, you need lots of love and support. The members of my church have been very helpful, and I had several healing sessions.'

What Should We Call It?

The term *Myalgic Encephalomyelitis* describes these main symptoms:

Myalgia = muscle pain
Encephalitis = affecting the brain
Myelitis = affecting the spinal cord and nerves

However, the term is not medically accurate, as 'itis' implies inflammation, and there is no evidence of active inflammation nor of infection of the brain or spinal cord, apart from maybe occasionally during the initial acute early stage.

Some doctors prefer to use the term *Post-viral Fatigue*

Syndrome, as it usually follows an apparent viral infection. There are many post-viral fatigue states, including fatigue for weeks after influenza, post-glandular fever debility, and debility for months following hepatitis. Myalgic Encephalomyelitis differs from other post-viral syndromes in its severity, the type of muscle fatigability, and chronicity.

An illness which has fatigue as its core symptom is now called *Chronic Fatigue Syndrome* in the USA and increasingly elsewhere in the world. Many doctors argue that this name is preferable since it does not imply any viral cause, nor involvement of the brain or muscles.

M.E. is the name commonly used by patients in the UK and recognized by the general population. Apart from anything else, 'M.E.' is easier to say than 'CFS' or 'PVFS'!

Chronic Fatigue Syndrome may be a disease-picture with various causes (a 'heterogenous condition'), and its definition is slightly different from that of M.E. Some people with CFS may have a post-viral syndrome. Some cases of post-viral fatigue have M.E.

Therefore, I regard the illness called Myalgic Encephalomyelitis as a post-viral fatigue syndrome, and also as one of a number of chronic fatigue syndromes; however, probably not all people diagnosed with Chronic Fatigue Syndrome have got M.E.

I address this book mainly to those with M.E., but also to people with any chronic fatigue syndrome for whom there is no clear diagnosis. When I quote research documents the terms M.E. or PVFS or CFS may be used, depending on the name used by the researchers.

Diagnosing M.E.

Myalgic Encephalomyelitis is recognized in a patient with these features:

1. Gross, abnormal muscle fatigue, which occurs after a

relatively small effort, and which may take days to be overcome. This is quite unlike any fatigue the patient has ever experienced before.

2. A variety of neuropsychiatric ('encephalitic') symptoms, most prominent being cognitive loss – of memory, concentration and comprehension – and disturbances of sensation.

3. Unpredictable variation in the severity of symptoms from week to week, day to day, even hour to hour.

4. A tendency for the symptoms to become chronic, i.e. lasting many months or years.

Other post-viral fatigue states do not continue for years. The diagnosis of M.E. should not be made unless the patient has the above features. Everyone feels tired when hit by a bout of influenza, a cold, or any infection. Most people who get a severe dose of influenza will be under-par for weeks, possibly months. Glandular fever and hepatitis are well known for the debility they cause, which persists for months. These conditions that require prolonged recovery are accurately called 'post-viral fatigue states'.

Many doctors say they find M.E. hard to diagnose, or to distinguish from a state of chronic depression. Some may still label the patient as malingering or hysterical. However, for most GPs, it is a condition that, once seen, is never forgotten. The post-exertional malaise after mild or moderate exertion is the most unique feature:

Typically, the patient tolerates the physical exertion reasonably well, and may even feel energized during and immediately after the exertion. However, 6–24 hours later the patients feel ill; the used muscle groups feel sore and weak . . . and most patients experience marked worsening of their fatigue, cognitive function, adenopathy, pharyngitis and fever. In our experience, this post-exertional malaise is unusual in healthy people, and in those with other diseases that have some resemblance to CFS.

(Komaroff 1991)

M.E. usually starts after an infection of some kind, with a sore throat, sore glands in the neck, fever, often pain in chest or neck, maybe vomiting and diarrhoea (gastric flu). There may be a period of apparent recovery, lasting a few weeks. This is followed by strange symptoms such as sudden collapse, vertigo, severe chest pain, abdominal symptoms, or recurrence of the flu symptoms.

At this stage, no one knows what is going on, and the patient may be put on antibiotics, sent to a cardiologist or other appropriate specialist, and given a few weeks off work. Complete rest for several weeks at this stage may lead to recovery.

But most people expect to be back to normal a few weeks after an infection. So the patient struggles back to work or school when the expected time-limit for recovery expires; then follow months of exhaustion, an inability to perform life's daily tasks, and a struggle to keep going, all the while believing that mind-over-matter will win – and it doesn't. The patient's symptoms get worse, he or she may be depressed or even suicidal. The patient cannot believe that this pathetic creature whose muscles don't work, whose brain is like porridge, who cries from pain and exhaustion after doing nearly nothing – maybe trying to get upstairs – can be the same fit and active individual he or she was before.

It is now realized that battling on and trying to get back to normal, in the acute stage, is *the worst possible thing to do*. This is why it is so crucial that people know about the existence of M.E., because if complete rest is allowed early on, before the illness becomes chronic, then there is a better chance of early recovery.

Unfortunately, most people expect a cure for nearly every illness nowadays. Old-fashioned principles of allowing the body to heal with rest, good food, fresh air and tranquillity have been forgotten; the majority of people only allow themselves one or two weeks to recover from a viral infection. If you had tuberculosis, or double pneumonia, or rheumatic fever, would you expect to be back working full-time after one or two weeks? Of course not.

It appears that a common mechanism that triggers off the development of M.E. is getting a viral infection while one is exhausted or highly stressed. However, some sufferers cannot pin-point the onset of their illness, and have gradually become more tired and ill over a period of time. On careful questioning, though, a history of having had an infection some time around the date of 'when were you last well?' will be remembered. The triggering infection may have seemed innocuous at the time. Occasionally the triggering incident is an immunization. It is easy to remember an attack of influenza; however, one of the most common viruses now implicated in M.E. (in the UK) is the group called 'enteroviruses', which may entail only a day or two of mild 'summer flu', or be symptomless and therefore overlooked.

Most of the earlier observations about M.E. have been based on patients studied in epidemics. In fact, M.E. occurs in both epidemic and endemic (isolated cases) form, and obviously a cluster of cases in one area will attract more attention than single, apparently unconnected cases scattered about. There is a history of recorded outbreaks going back to 1934, when an epidemic of what seemed at first to be poliomyelitis was reported in Los Angeles. This was the first of no less than 52 recorded outbreaks from various parts of the world, up to the present time.

A diagnosis of 'neurasthenia' was popularized by an American psychiatrist, George Beard, in 1869, for a condition with some resemblances to Chronic Fatigue Syndrome today. The diagnosis became popular and fashionable, and probably some of the patients labelled neurasthenic had M.E. But the diagnosis came to include so many non-specific symptoms that it fell out of favour. However, it exists in the *International*

Classification of Disease, having now a narrower definition than Beard's original one.

Florence Nightingale became ill after returning from her heroic work in the Crimean war, and spent years housebound and too exhausted to speak to more than one visitor at a time. She certainly had something like M.E.; she also had a high-risk career.

The Los Angeles Epidemic

The Los Angeles epidemic (1934) had features which initially resembled poliomyelitis. At the Los Angeles County General Hospital 198 staff became ill. The main features which differed from those of polio were:

- Lack of severe muscle wasting, as would be expected in polio.
- Longer-lasting muscle pain and tenderness, and sensory symptoms.
- Memory lapses, loss of concentration, sleep disturbances, emotional instability, and inability to walk a short distance without fatigue.

Over 50 per cent of the staff were still unable to work six months after the peak of the epidemic.

The Royal Free Epidemic

The best known outbreak of M.E. in Britain took place in 1955, when nearly 300 members of hospital staff at London's Royal Free Hospital developed what was obviously an infectious illness, over a period of four-and-a-half months. Of the ill hospital staff, 255 had to be admitted to hospital, and yet only 12 of the patients who were already in hospital during the epidemic developed the disease. It is probable that the patients were protected from developing the muscle and neurological symptoms of M.E. because they were resting in bed, whereas the hospital staff were busy and physically active when they became infected. In this way, M.E. behaves like polio in an epidemic.

The clinical features of this epidemic among Royal Free Hospital staff (doctors, nurses, ancillary workers, and administrative personnel) were as follows:

- Malaise, headache, sore throat, abdominal pain, nausea, enlarged glands.
  These were the initial symptoms, and they fluctuated for several days.
- Severe pain in the back, neck, limbs, or between ribs; dizziness or vertigo.
  These symptoms developed after a few days.
- Neurological signs and symptoms developed by week three or four. 74 per cent of patients showed evidence of involvement of the central nervous system. Symptoms included double vision, difficulty swallowing, paralysis of the face, weakness of arms and legs, twitching or spasms of muscles, and bladder problems.
- Spontaneous pains with muscle tenderness and weak limbs were common features.

There are some of these Royal Free hospital staff who still suffer today from the illness, which was called *epidemic neuromyesthenia*. The infectious agent responsible was not isolated. A full account of the many outbreaks since 1934 has been written by Dr Melvin Ramsay in his book *The Saga of Royal Free Disease*.

The Iceland Epidemic

The outbreak in Iceland in 1948–9 is very interesting, because in 1955 there was a poliomyelitis epidemic on the island, which did not produce cases in the districts where the epidemic neuromyesthenia had occurred in 1948. This implied that whatever virus was responsible for the M.E. provided immunity against polio.

Common Features

The clinical features of many outbreaks world-wide (for example Los Angeles 1934, Iceland, Adelaide 1949–51,

Coventry 1953, Durban 1955, which all corresponded with epidemics of poliomyelitis) had certain features in common:

- An obvious infection
- Involvement of the central nervous system
- Prolonged fluctuating course
- Marked muscle fatigability
- Exhaustion

A proportion of patients were left physically incapacitated for many years.

The Symptoms of M.E.

In a recent questionnaire (one of several) of people who gave a typical history and had the cardinal M.E. symptoms, the following were the various symptoms given, in rough order of frequency:

Made worse by exercise – 100 per cent
Exhaustion and severe malaise – 85 per cent
Muscle weakness after using muscle, lasting days
Muscle pain – commonest in back of shoulders, upper
  arms, and thighs
Blurring of vision – sometimes actual double vision
Sensation of pins and needles, or numbness
Loss of concentration
Headache
Muscle twitching
Speech difficulties – e.g. using the wrong word, or
  being unable to come up with the word needed
Poor circulation – cold hands and feet
Pain in the back of neck
Abnormal sweating – often with a sour smell
Impairment of memory, especially for recent events
Breathing difficulty – sensation of lack of air
Extreme sensitivity to sound – called 'hyperacusis'
Noises in ears – called 'tinnitus'

Sleep disturbance
Palpitations, and/or racing heartbeat
Difficulty standing for any time – (classic symptom of M.E.)
Vivid or bad dreams
Joint pains – which may move from joint to joint
Feeling 'spaced out', disorientated
Depression
Loss of interest in sex
Nausea
Chest pains
Emotional lability – crying easily, rapid mood change
Constipation or diarrhoea
Recurrent sore throats
Enlarged or painful lymph glands
Altered sense of taste and/or smell
Difficulty with balance and/or true vertigo
Difficulty walking, or walking having to be limited to very short distances
Panic attacks
Poor temperature control
Poor co-ordination – clumsiness
Pallor when ill – quite common
Poor bladder control
Skin very sensitive to touch
Spontaneous bruising, skin rashes
Great thirst

These symptoms are not present all of the time, but the features common to all are:

Exhaustion, and symptoms made worse by exercise.

Age and Sex Distribution – from Questionnaire

Male : Female		1 : 3
Age: Under 20		3.5%
20–29		15.0%
30–39		28.5%
40–49		23.0%

| 50–59 | 20.0% |
| Over 60 | 10.0% |

Duration of Illness – At Time of Response

Less than 2 years	35.0%
Over 2 years	65.0%
Over 5 years	33.0%
Over 10 years	12.0%
Over 20 years	4.0%

Various other studies have produced slightly different figures, but it seems that, from the date of onset of the illness one has a 30 per cent chance of still having symptoms of M.E. after five years. Of course many of the chronic sufferers may not be as badly affected after five years as they were at the outset. Also, most will not have been continuously ill, but will have had remissions and relapses.

Another way of predicting the future is this: If you are in the first year of the illness, the chances of getting better are:

50 per cent in 2 years,
60 per cent in 5 years, and
90 per cent in 10 years.

However, 'better' is an inexact word. What most patients mean by 'better' is being able to live a nearly normal life for much of the time, but avoiding strenuous exercise. I know of very few people who had typical post-viral M.E. who have returned 100 per cent to their pre-illness fitness level.

Of the long list of symptoms given above, most occur in many other diseases, and are non-specific. Are there 'typical' M.E. symptoms?

• History of a virus infection before onset
• Exhaustion out of all proportion to the effort made
• Symptoms which suggest a chronic or recurrent infec-

tion – intermittent fever, tender lymph nodes, sore throat.

• Muscle problems:
  Muscle weakness brought on after minimal effort, which may take several days or weeks to go away.
  Inability to stand – the legs shake and ache after standing for a short time, and the patient has to sit down, on the ground if necessary.
  Inability to hold arms up – cannot hang up washing, difficulty carrying bags or even holding telephone receiver.
  Aching back or neck if sitting in unsupporting chair.
  Intermittent blurring of vision – due to fatigue of the eye muscle which alters the focus (ciliary muscle); or of the muscles which keep the eyes moving together to give a clear single image – failure of these may produce double vision.
  Aching in the face after chewing; inability to write for long.
  General muscle tenderness, with some acutely sensitive local spots.
  Note that problems arise from *sustained* muscle use; the muscle function may be normal to start with, e.g. in the morning, but pain and weakness develop after using the muscles for a short time. Slow walking may be easier than standing. The muscles most commonly affected are the girdle muscles – the back of the shoulders, the buttocks and thighs.

• 'Encephalitic', or brain symptoms:
  Poor concentration – typically concentration cannot be sustained for long, whether you are listening to the radio, reading, or having a conversation.
  Poor memory – forgetting the name of someone you know well, forgetting what has just been said, not knowing where you are or why you are there (e.g. if driving, being totally disorientated and lost, though in a familiar place).

Nominal aphasia – inability to find the word for something.

Muddled or even slurred speech when tired.

Hypersensitivity to sound – maybe so severe that voices, radio, clocks ticking are all unbearable.

Hypersensitivity to light, also to touch – e.g. clothes hurt if they touch your skin. Maybe tingling sensations, or pins and needles.

Transient blurred or double vision.

Increased sense of smell, or smelling bizarre odours that cannot be traced to their source.

Nightmares, sleep disturbance, deficiency in certain levels of sleep.

- Autonomic nervous system (controls all involuntary body functions – also part of brain disturbance):

    Sudden racing heartbeat, or palpitations.

    Profuse sweating, even when cold.

    Pallor – often an ashen grey colour – at onset of feeling ill.

    Poor temperature regulation.

    Poor circulation to hands and feet – maybe only affecting one side.

    Alternating diarrhoea or constipation.

    Poor blood-sugar control.

    Difficulty passing urine, or incontinence.

- Acute neurological events happen in only a few patients:

    'Primary seizures (7 per cent), acute profound ataxia (6 per cent), focal weakness (5 per cent), transient loss of vision (4 per cent). These were mostly during the first year of the illness.' (Komaroff 1991)

Other Symptoms

- Sudden mood changes, untypical of the person.
- Development of new allergies – particularly to chemicals and some foods.
- Difficulty breathing – especially at night – the 'I wake

up feeling I cannot get enough oxygen' symptom.
• Joint pains, sometimes with swelling.
• Prostatic symptoms in men.

The Progression of the Illness

The natural progression of the illness is a slow improvement, *if proper rest is allowed*. Most M.E. people relapse because they are active by nature, and as soon as they start to feel better they do too much, then become ill again.

Main Causes of Relapse

• Physical exercise beyond the safe limit for the day.
• Mental overwork, particularly intense concentration, e.g. studying for exams.
• Developing another infection.
• Hormonal changes – such as during menstruation, or after childbirth.
• Major stresses – moving house, divorce, bereavement, etc.
• Exposure to chemicals – e.g. new paint.
• Extreme change of climate.
• Winter – not only the cold, but the lack of daylight.
• Surgery, anaesthetics, dental treatment.

There are a small number of sufferers who do not seem to have any remissions, and who gradually deteriorate, but these are relatively few. More often the illness fluctuates, with relapses and remissions occurring, sometimes quite unpredictably. This is one of the features of M.E. that makes it so hard to assess clinically, especially in any trial of treatment. The marked variations in symptoms and in the degree of illness felt by a sufferer also leads to disbelief on the part of family, friends and one's doctor. People find it hard to accept that you have a genuine illness if they see you in a wheelchair one week, and walking the next. What they don't see is that you can still only walk a short way, and they don't observe your collapse when you get home!

Chronic Fatigue Syndrome

In order for this condition to be recognizable, and also to improve the basis for clinical research, a working case definition was required – one which could be accepted world-wide. In the USA, a number of physicians have together drawn up the criteria for a case definition of Chronic Fatigue Syndrome. Another name used in the USA is Chronic Fatigue and Immune Dysfunction Syndrome – CFIDS.

Major Criteria for CFS

1. *New* onset of persistent or relapsing debilitating fatigue, or easy fatigability in a person with no such previous symptom, that does not resolve with bed rest and is severe enough to reduce daily activity below 50 per cent of what it was before the illness, for at least six months.
2. Other clinical conditions which could cause this fatigue must be excluded by history, examination, and appropriate investigations.

Both of these criteria need to be met for a diagnosis of CFS to be given.

Minor Criteria

The following symptoms must have persisted or recurred over six months, and have developed at or after the onset of fatigue.

- Mild fever or chills
- Sore throat
- Painful lymph glands
- Muscle weakness
- Muscle pain or tenderness

- Prolonged (24 hours or more) fatigue following a level of exercise that previously caused no problems
- Headaches different in type to the kind experienced before the illness
- Joint pains
- Neuropsychologic complaints (encephalitic) – one or more of the following:
    light sensitivity
    blind spots in vision
    loss of memory
    irritability
    confusion
    poor concentration
    inability to think clearly
    depression
- Sleep disturbance

Physical Criteria

These symptoms have to have been observed by a doctor at least twice, and to have occurred at least a month apart:

- Low-grade fever
- Inflamed throat
- Palpable or tender lymph nodes in neck or armpits

At least eight symptom criteria need to be fulfilled; or at least six symptom plus two physical criteria.

In the USA, chronic Epstein Barr virus was thought to be the cause of M.E./CFS – which used to be called CEBV syndrome. There is also more emphasis in the USA on the fever, sore throat, and tender lymph gland symptoms. In the UK most cases are probably triggered by an enterovirus, and the clinical picture, with the muscle symptoms predominant, is more specific than that for CFS. I believe that a diagnosis of M.E. should be reserved for patients with the clinical features listed on page 21, and that M.E. is probably just one type of chronic fatigue syndrome.

In 1988 Dr A. Lloyd and others of New South Wales, Australia, developed a set of diagnostic criteria after reviewing 100 patients, for a diagnosis of chronic fatigue syndrome (the term they prefer to M.E.):

1. Chronic or relapsing fatigue, made worse by very minor exercise, causing disruption of daily life, and of over six months' duration;
2. Neuropsychiatric dysfunction, including impairment of concentration, short-term memory loss; and/or
3. Evidence of abnormal cell mediated immunity.

They consider the following findings supportive to the above three main criteria:

Muscle pain, joint pain, headaches, depression, tinnitus, paraesthesiae (abnormal sensations), sleep disturbance, tender lymph glands, sore throats.

These observations, coupled with the laboratory evidence of disordered immune function in many patients, suggests that something triggers off the disease, most commonly a viral infection, in a person whose immune system is already damaged in some way. It is possible that some as yet unidentified infectious agent – call it agent X – affects the immune system, and this together with an inherited susceptibility allows either a common viral illness to trigger the illness, or a latent infection to be reactivated.

Current contenders for agent X include the recently discovered HHV-6, (human herpes virus 6) and a retrovirus related to HTLV-2 (the one implicated in HIV/AIDS), but these claims are not yet substantiated. Or could agent X be the damage caused by global pollution on an increasing scale? This might explain why the incidence of M.E. and CFS seems to be increasing, although the illness is not new.

Incidence of M.E./CFS

There is great need for careful epidemiological surveys to establish the true incidence of M.E. in the UK. In

Australia (Lloyd and others, 1990) a study of a population of 114,000 found 42 cases of chronic fatigue syndrome which fulfilled strict diagnostic criteria. This gives a prevalence of 37.1 cases per 100,000 (for Multiple Sclerosis this figure is 36.5 per 100,000, in New South Wales). In 75 per cent of cases the onset of M.E. followed an acute 'viral' illness.

The Controversy – is M.E. a Disease, or All in the Mind?

In 1970, two psychiatrists at the Middlesex Hospital, London, produced two papers in the *British Medical Journal*: 'Royal Free Epidemic of 1955: a reconsideration', and 'Concept of Benign Myalgic Encephalomyelitis'.

In these papers they gave their reasons for considering that the Royal Free epidemic of 1955 had been an outbreak of mass hysteria, and that other outbreaks in the world also had features of hysteria. They admitted that those outbreaks which showed a resemblance to poliomyelitis probably weren't cases of mass hysteria, but took no account of the clinical features of those affected.

In spite of the fact that there were obvious flaws in their reasoning – such as the signs of infection and neurological involvement, which could not be hysterically-produced – this hypothesis about M.E. given by McEvedy and Beard was taken up by the media, and has unfortunately been accepted without question by many within the medical profession since that time.

The damage done to people who have had this illness, both those of the Royal Free outbreak and others since, has been incalculable. Of course it is much more convenient to label the condition as hysterical; there is then no need to research the illness, patients can be ordered to pull their socks up and go back to work, and those who have no experience of the devastating symptoms can rejoice in being far too well-balanced to get 'that sort of complaint'.

Thanks to the tireless efforts of certain doctors, who never doubted the reality of the disease, in the last few years evidence has emerged, through various research studies, of the real and organic nature of the illness. Special credit is due to Dr Melvin Ramsay, who was consultant in infectious diseases at the Royal Free Hospital at the time of the 1955 outbreak, and who devoted a large part of his long working life to striving for the recognition of and research into M.E. Sadly Dr Ramsay died in March 1990; he is greatly missed by the many people he helped during his long battle to get M.E. recognized. During the last two years, many soundly-based research projects have got under way; some of these are discussed in Chapter 3.

Not only some doctors, but also patients themselves have campaigned for better recognition and understanding. The M.E. Association, founded in 1976, and the more recently formed M.E. Action, have provided support and information to sufferers, and have worked to educate doctors, politicians and those working in the social services about the nature of the illness and its debilitating effects. What we still lack is an accurate figure for the incidence of M.E. in the UK population.

It is salutary to note that about 20 years ago, unfortunate victims of that most disabling condition Multiple Sclerosis were labelled as neurotic or hysterical. Now MS is recognized, and yet its diagnosis is largely a clinical one; there is still no single specific test for MS which is widely available.

Modern medicine relies increasingly on laboratory tests and X-rays for diagnosis, and less and less on each patient's history. A problem for doctors trying to evaluate a patient's history lies in defining the main symptom – *fatigue*. This complaint may come from someone who 'feels tired a lot, doesn't feel like getting up in the morning'. Fatigue may also be a complaint of someone who collapses and feels very ill after minimal exertion, but who has a previous history of great energy and activity. So 'fatigue' can mean many things . . .

This confusion of the symptom of 'chronic fatigue' with M.E. and CFS may be seen in some well-argued recent papers published in the last two years in medical journals, which tend to emphasize the psychiatric symptoms of chronic fatigue. Depression is a symptom, not a disease itself, and is frequently a prominent and disabling part of M.E. It is also a common symptom in other organic brain disorders, including MS, Alzheimer's disease, and Parkinson's disease; reactive depression can develop in any chronic illness. Psychiatric symptoms in M.E. should be treated where appropriate – but do not in themselves mean that the disease is psychological in origin.

Much excellent research is being done, looking at the evidence of persistent virus and at immune dysfunction. However, every time some new evidence of the organic nature of M.E. appears, someone writes an indignant letter pointing out flaws in the research, and providing a psychological explanation for the results.

Here is an extract from an article called 'Chronic fatigue, viruses and depression' – note the use of the term chronic fatigue, which could be interpreted as meaning the same thing as M.E.:

> It is important to recognize that, in a society where M.E. is portrayed as a mysterious, rather glamorous, and disabling illness, people who have acquired this diagnosis may obtain attention and sympathy from friends and relatives, and perhaps also a justification for not fulfilling career ambitions or coping with the demands of everyday life. They may therefore lead less unhappy lives with their symptoms and their diagnosis than they could do otherwise.

This person's view is not based on any scientific study of numbers of ill people, it is an unfounded opinion.

There are of course a number of people who have needs that are satisfied by the invalid role, to be found in any chronic illness group. But to print this biased opinion, in a way that seems to apply to M.E. in particular, can only have far-reaching, harmful effects on ill people who are struggling to cope.

One of the characteristics of people with genuine M.E. is that they are highly motivated, frustrated by not being physically able to do things, and try by any means to get better. The loss of careers, breakdown of marriages, loss of ability to function in nearly every aspect of life – these devastating results of the disease cannot lead to 'less unhappy lives'. In addition, many people with M.E. get neither sympathy nor support from family or friends.

However, if M.E. is portrayed as nothing more than being chronically tired, then misconceptions such as that quoted above are bound to persist.

> Fatigue is a common complaint of patients presenting at general medical practice. Many such patients probably are suffering from a primary psychiatric illness. A few may have a well-recognized organic cause of chronic fatigue, such as hidden malignancy, thyroid disease, anaemia or other illness. Probably only a few of many patients seeking medical care for chronic fatigue have M.E./CFS.
>
> *(Komaroff 1991)*

It is therefore very important for doctors to understand the difference between the complaint of chronic fatigue, and the features of M.E.

In case any of you doubt that the McEvedy and Beard (hysteria) diagnosis is still around, let me relate the account of a mother's difficulty when her daughter became ill:

'My daughter, aged 11, fell ill with a virus which was going round her school. She did not recover properly, and for months she kept on having swollen glands, a sore throat, and a slight fever. After eight months she was keen to go to school, but some days she would fade out by mid-morning and have to come home. If she tried any sports or gym she collapsed. She was referred to a paediatrician, who did blood tests and found nothing wrong. We then took her to another children's doctor, privately; he said he could find nothing wrong, and that she should be encouraged to go to school (which she was keen to do). We took her to see a consultant rheumatologist, because she had these awful pains in her muscles and legs, and he told us that she just needed to exercise and get fit!

'Then I saw an article in the *Telegraph* which described her condition exactly. We were so relieved to find out what was wrong. I went back to see the private specialist and showed him the newspaper article, saying – ''Look at this, our daughter has got post-viral Fatigue Syndrome.'' He just dismissed it, and said ''That is Royal Free Disease, that's been proven to be hysteria.''

'We were upset and angry. I knew she was ill and not putting it on. The trouble was that we needed a doctor to give a diagnosis so that she could rest from school if unwell, and be excused from having to do any sport.'

It was at this stage that this worried mother told me the story, and fortunately I was able to put her in touch with a knowledgeable GP, who recognized the illness with no difficulty. Happily the girl is now gradually improving, and a year after having the virus is able to go to school, provided she does not exercise.

But here were *three* specialists, all in one small city, who could not recognize that this child was ill, in part because they relied on blood tests rather than her history.

Chapter 2

The Immune System

The immune system is mentioned quite often in this book and in many others about health, so for non-medical readers, here is a very simplified description.

The body is constantly invaded by 'foreign' substances. The immune system is the protective mechanism which prevents damage to the body by invaders. Any thing which is 'non-self' is recognized as foreign, and is normally disposed of or made harmless by a healthy immune system.

The invader may be:

Microbes – viruses, bacteriae, yeasts,
Parasites – worms, malaria, amoeba, giardia, etc.
Foreign tissues – e.g. transplants
Poisons – this includes alcohol, drugs, chemical additives in food, air and water, smoke, as well as other poisons
Cancer cells
Dust, pollens, moulds.

It is the defensive reaction against a potentially harmful thing that produces symptoms. For example, the pain of a boil is not caused by the germs in it, but results from the swelling and increased blood flow to the area. If there was not this local painful reaction, the infection would not be sealed off and attacked, but could spread throughout the body, with serious results. Similarly, the fever and malaise that are features of the common cold are not caused by the virus, but by the chemicals produced by the immune system doing battle with the virus. In fact people whose immune system is not efficient may not have much of a fever when they have an infection.

The army the body has for its defence consists of white blood cells with different divisions, and their weapons, i.e. the substances made by white cells which help them deal with the invaders.

The white blood cells are made in the bone marrow. They are much less numerous than red blood cells (red blood cells carry oxygen round the body), but are essential to life.

The types of white blood cell are:

1. Polymorphs – their name means 'changing shape' – also called granulocytes, because they contain granules which release chemicals which are poisonous to microbes. They are relatively large, and their main job is scavenging. They are highly mobile, and rush in large numbers to the site of an injury or an infection. They can engulf a bacterium by changing shape, and once inside produce chemicals which digest the germ. They are found in large numbers in pus.

2. Macrophages – large scavengers of dead tissue and foreign particles, also involved in immune reactions to destroy cells. They can produce inflammatory chemicals that cause pain, swelling, and redness in tissues. Many microbial infections that do not respond to conventional antibiotics involve microbial infestation of macrophages – e.g. tuberculosis – in which cases the infected macrophages release chemicals that can destroy surrounding tissue. Macrophages, after ingesting a foreign particle (such as a virus) can also activate T-cells.

3. Lymphocytes – two main kinds:
    B lymphocytes, matured in the Bursal or lymph tissues, and
    T lymphocytes, matured in the Thymus gland.
These are also called T-cells and B-cells.

B Lymphocytes

B lymphocytes produce *antibodies* (immunoglobulins) to microbes and to their toxins. An antibody is specific for the antigen – *antigen* means the thing which has stimulated the lymphocyte to make an antibody. A second exposure to the antigen induces a greater production of antibody to it, because the recipe for that particular antibody is stored on the surface of 'memory' cells – another function of white cells – and on recognition of the antigen, the B lymphocytes are stimulated to make the antibody.

This how immunization works, and also why one becomes immune to certain diseases – e.g. measles – after one attack. These antibodies, or Immunoglobulins, are very large molecules of protein and are classified into groups, called IgA, IgM, IgG, and IgE, and then into subclasses, e.g. IgG3 – which is thought to play a major role in virus neutralization.

T Lymphocytes

There are also further subdivisions of T lymphocytes, or T-cells. There are *helper* cells, which help the B lymphocytes to produce antibodies and the polymorphs and macrophages to kill or engulf foreign matter. And when a battle with some invader is over, the *suppressor* cells stop the reaction. T-cells are given numbers; more are being discovered each year – e.g. CD4, CD8, CD56.

There are also *natural killer* – NK – cells, which destroy infected cells.

T-cells produce various chemicals called *cytokines* (or lymphokines). Names of cytokines include interferon, interleukin 1, and interleukin 2. They help in the task of killing infected cells, and a raised level in the blood suggests an ongoing viral infection. Cytokines also control the synthesis of immunoglobulins by the B-cells. Cytokines cause inflammation, and are involved in allergic responses; they are responsible for the unpleasant symptoms of influenza – fever, aching, headache, shivering, weepiness.

All white blood cells circulate in the blood and in all tissues of the body, on patrol for invaders, and can move to where they are needed.

The T lymphocytes are active against viruses, as well as helping B-cells with their work. Viruses can only survive and replicate inside living cells, so T-cells have to be able to kill the cells invaded by the virus.

Anything that

a) reduces the number of white cells
b) reduces their mobility
c) weakens their killing ability

will weaken the body's defence against a viral infection.

In some interreactions between antigen (a foreign agent) and the immune system, antigen-antibody 'immune complexes' are formed. In this and some other reactions, certain proteins called *complements* are used up. Other proteins may become greater in amount, e.g. C-reactive proteins. I mention this because such names come up in accounts of immunology research in M.E.

The study of immunology is relatively new in medical science; I doubt that many doctors other than immunologists really understand the immune system in depth. The above is a *very* simplified overview, and I have not attempted any proper descriptions of how the lymphocytes and cytokines work.

Chapter 3

What Causes M.E.?
I – Virus and Muscle Research

To give you a flavour of the current ideas about what causes M.E. and the Chronic Fatigue Syndrome, I can do no better than to quote directly the theories of three researchers, each of whom has seen and investigated many hundreds of patients:

> Post-viral fatigue syndrome is a metabolic disorder, caused by persistent virus infection and associated with defective immunoregulation.
>
> *(Prof P. O. Behan, 1985)*

> The condition (M.E.) appears to be a rare complication, mainly in non-immune adults, of a widespread often asymptomatic childhood infection. The group of viruses most consistently associated with M.E. are the non-polio enteroviruses – including Coxsackie and Echoviruses.
>
> When the host immune response is ineffective, viral parasitism leads to mitochondrial damage with resultant energy deficits at cellular level.
>
> *(Dr E. Dowsett, 1990)*

> It is presumed that CFIDS (CFS) is a cytokine-mediated illness, virally induced, in genetically susceptible individuals. [CFIDS=Chronic Fatigue and Immune Dysfunction Syndrome, a term for CFS also used in the USA.]
>
> *(Dr Jay Goldstein, 1990)*

Research has been done into various aspects of M.E., carried out in differing medical specialities:

Virology, and effects of viruses in the body
Muscle abnormalities
Immunology

Red blood cell abnormalities
Neurology, brain involvement
Psychology, psychiatry

Viruses and M.E.

The Case for Enteroviruses

In a small town on the Hudson River in New York State in the late 1940s, a new virus was isolated from children with a disease that resembled poliomyelitis. The virus was named Coxsackie, after the town. It is now known that Coxsackie viruses are members of a group called *enteroviruses*, which include polioviruses and live in the human intestine. Enteroviruses can affect many tissues, but have a particular affinity for the central nervous system and muscles.

In two outbreaks of M.E. in Scotland in 1983, there were significant numbers of patients who had higher levels of antibodies to Coxsackie B virus than were found in the general population.

In a further report of patients with symptoms of M.E. in a west Scotland general practice (1984), nearly half had high Coxsackie B antibody levels. In this same practice, 55 per cent of those with Coxsackie infection were still ill after one year, nearly all having persistently high antibody levels. So it was probable that Coxsackie B virus was responsible for several outbreaks of an M.E.-like illness in Scotland.

The most comprehensive summary of the role of enterovirus infection in M.E. can be found in the paper: 'Myalgic encephalomyelitis – a persistent enteroviral infection?' (Dowsett, 1990)

The human enterovirus family comprises about 70 species, including: polioviruses, Coxsackie A and B, echoviruses, hepatitis A and B, sub-groups of these species, and others. Records exist of enterovirus disease going back to 2000 BC.

Now that a polio vaccine has reduced the incidence of paralytic polio, the non-polio enteroviruses are becoming more important in causing human disease. History has shown that enteroviruses have a great capacity to start new syndromes and new epidemics.

Enteroviruses are known to cause many clinical conditions; examples of enteroviral illnesses are:

Respiratory infections
Gastroenteritis
Hepatitis
Meningitis and encephalitis
Poliomyelitis
Bornholm's disease – (severe chest pain due to involvement of the muscles between the ribs)
Myocarditis and pericarditis
Hand, foot and mouth disease, and other skin conditions
Conjunctivitis
Pancreatitis and juvenile onset diabetes, and
Myalgic Encephalomyelitis

Enteroviruses are known to affect muscle and nerve particularly. The two main tissues affected in M.E. are muscle and nerve; enteroviruses are said to be 'myotropic and neurotropic.'

Enteroviruses are spread from the faeces of those infected, via sewage, rivers, estuaries, beaches and agriculture, to reinfect humans in drinking water and food. They are easily picked up on beach and water holidays; by hospital workers from bedpans and other equipment; by those who work with young children – who frequently harbour enteroviruses without signs of illness – and land and water workers. Most enteroviral infections do not cause any obvious illness. Enteroviruses are not killed in the process of 'treating' sewage before it enters the sea.

In several outbreaks of M.E., patients were initially thought to have polio (e.g. Los Angeles 1934, Iceland

1948), and health authorities thought a polio epidemic had started, until it became clear that the illness, although resembling poliomyelitis, had some different features. One aspect in which M.E. behaved like polio was that *those who were most physically active when they contracted the infection were most likely to develop muscle weakness.*

In a follow-up study of M.E. cases from a Glasgow college (Durndell, 1989), out of the 31 patients, 12 had been runners pre-illness, whereas only 2 of the 25 healthy controls were runners.

Evidence that enteroviruses are present in a sizable number of M.E. patients resulted from the work of Professor James Mowbray and his colleagues at St Mary's Medical School, London (Mowbray, 1988).

It is difficult to detect virus in the stools because it is bound with antibody, so a method was devised which would detect enterovirus-group-protein in the blood. This protein, called VP1 polypeptide, is common to all members of the enterovirus family. VP1 was detected in the blood of 51 per cent of the tested M.E. patients.

This VP1 test has since been carried out on many more patients with clinical features of M.E., and is positive in about 60 per cent of the cases. If positive, it simply means that there is active enterovirus in the body, but does not identify which one, because the virus protein is common to all of them.

However, the test is also positive in a number of healthy people, and reflects the amount of that enteroviral infection in a community at any time. Enteroviral infections are extremely common, and frequently asymptomatic. The VP1 test, though useful in giving supporting evidence to the diagnosis of M.E. if consistently positive over a period of months, is not now included in routine tests on a patient suspected of having M.E. – it is too non-specific. What distinguishes those with M.E. from others carrying enterovirus is their *abnormal response* to the virus.

The Iceland Research – Akureyri, 40 Years Later
(Hyde and Bergman, 1991)

In Iceland in 1948, the outbreak of an illness that resembled polio but was epidemic myalgic encephalomyelitis, was centred around a small community at Akureyri. Dr B. M. Hyde from Canada has studied some people who fell ill during the 1948 outbreak and are still alive.

Ten people, now aged between 58 and 84, were interviewed, examined and had blood tests performed. Only two out of the ten had made a complete recovery, even after 40 years. They had all had features typical of myalgic encephalomyelitis when they were ill. One had fallen ill in 1955, the others in 1948. Records indicated that the disease became endemic after the 1948 outbreak, so sporadic cases would have continued for years.

Eight out of the ten had a positive enterovirus VP1 test; the two who were negative were the two who had made a complete recovery. Those people who had not made a complete recovery all had some degree of chronic handicap, although they all thought they had made a good recovery. On psychological assessment, none of the ten showed any signs of neurosis or hysteria; they had all achieved satisfying lives or careers in spite of varying levels of disability.

This evidence points to a persistent virus being involved in M.E. Here in Iceland were people who had fallen ill 40 years ago, who all conformed to the features of M.E. syndrome; after 40 years, eight out of ten still had enterovirus in their blood, also persisting disabilities, yet had successfully overcome their handicaps of chronic illness.

Effects of Enteroviruses in the Body
Enteroviruses are known to infect muscle, including heart muscle, the nerves and the brain. They may also infect endocrine glands (e.g. the pancreas, leading to

diabetes). Enterovirus RNA (ribonucleic acid) has been identified in muscle cells of M.E. patients (see page 55). Certain strains may affect the heart, others the brain.

> Myocarditis and other cardiac problems, e.g. pericarditis, occur in up to 30 per cent patients with M.E., depending on whether the virus is a cardiogenic strain. This condition may persist long after recovery from the initial infection, in the form of auto-immune myocarditis. The connection between enteroviruses and cardiac disease has been documented for over 30 years.
>
> *(Personal communication from Dr E. Dowsett)*

The conducting tissue may also be affected, causing irregular heartbeat.

Brain Findings in M.E. Patients

Enterovirus can infect brain tissue. Dr J. Richardson, a GP from Newcastle, recovered brains from three M.E. patients who committed suicide. Prof. J. Mowbray was able to demonstrate enteroviral protein in the cortex of each brain. Using a dye that was specific for enterovirus, staining was observed around small blood vessels, and in glial (nerve) cells. Each patient had been ill for at least two years with an illness typical of post-viral onset M.E. Control brain specimens were entirely free of enterovirus in both the brain and bloodstream. In at least one victim, there was a high blood level of antibody to Coxsackie B, and a positive VP1. [This information comes from a presentation made by Dr Richardson at a symposium on M.E., June 1989, London].

Arthropathy in M.E.

Pain with or without swelling of joints is a well-recognized complication of M.E. It may be caused in several ways:

A direct viral infection (as in rubella). Enteroviruses have been isolated from joints of M.E. patients.

Immune complexes (found in 60 per cent of the patients in one survey) may settle in joints and cause symptoms of inflammation.

People with a genetic tendency to get arthritis will relapse if they get a viral infection (e.g. rheumatoid arthritis, which is not caused by M.E., flares up with a virus.)

(Personal communication from Dr E. Dowsett)

The Epstein Barr Virus

Chronic fatigue syndrome was known as Chronic Epstein Barr Virus disease (CEBV) in the USA until recently. The EB virus is a member of the herpes family, a different family from enteroviruses. Herpes viruses are 'DNA viruses', while enteroviruses are 'RNA viruses' – DNA and RNA being the two types of molecules which carry the genetic codes for reproduction. EB virus is best known for causing infectious mononucleosis, known (incorrectly) as glandular fever in the UK.

EB viral DNA has been found in 20 per cent of the patients in Dr Archard's muscle study which detected enterovirus RNA (see page 55), but not in the same muscle biopsy specimens.

Glandular fever is well known for the prolonged debility that persists for months after the acute infection. Most people have been infected with the EB virus by the age of 30, usually with few symptoms; only in a few is the infection severe enough to cause glandular fever. If you look for evidence of past EB infection, you will find it in about 95 per cent of people, with or without M.E.

Testing for active infection with EB virus requires special tests (see Appendix B). If these tests indicate an active, present EB virus infection in someone with symptoms of M.E., what has probably happened is that a latent EB virus that has hidden in some body cells for many years has become reactivated, causing active or persistent infection. The EB virus can hide in surface cells of the nose or throat, and in B lymphocytes for years. Depression of the immune system (maybe from another virus) allows it to flare up.

Two researchers, Prof. J. Mowbray (London) and Prof. J. C. Murdoch (New Zealand) found 20 per cent and 19 per cent (respectively) blood samples positive for active EB virus from patients with M.E. It is possible that other viruses which can remain latent in the body may be reactivated, and appear to trigger M.E.

A newly identified virus, *HHV-6 – human herpes virus 6* has been considered as being involved in M.E. However, researchers in Australia (Wakefield, 1988) found no difference in incidence of HHV-6 between M.E. patients and healthy controls. By one year of age, about 60 per cent of children have antibodies to HHV-6, showing that it is very common and acquired early in life.

However, Dr Josephs and others (1991) have found raised antibody titres to HHV-6 in six out of seven patients with CFS. Cell cultures produced HHV-6 DNA in three of the patients. The authors suggest that HHV-6 may be contributory to the pathogenesis of CFS. However, it may represent a reactivated virus, and not be the main cause (see page 60).

Another proposed culprit is a newly discovered retrovirus. Dr Elaine DeFreitas of Philadelphia (1990) presented a paper at a congress of neuropathology in Japan. She told how 23 out of 30 (77 per cent) blood samples from CFS patients contained virus particles that resembled those of HTLV 1 and HTLV 2 (retroviruses). The viral particles were detected using polymerase chain reaction (see page 55). In a separate study, antibodies to HTLV 1 and 2 were found in 50 per cent of the blood samples from these 30 patients. Dr DeFreitas' research team are now trying to isolate the virus. This discovery has not so far been repeated by other researchers, and at present the role of retroviruses in chronic fatigue syndromes is unknown.

A Persistent Viral Fatigue Syndrome?

It now seems possible, certainly in M.E. people with enterovirus, that part of the virus is persisting inside cells, and is interfering with the cells' functions. This is indeed a feature of *persistent virus infections*, which are recognized increasingly as being involved in several chronic illnesses of unknown cause. In acute viral infections which clear up, there is a reaction by the body's defence system; this results in the death of cells that are infected by the virus, and prevents the virus from infecting other cells. Therefore the virus, which can only replicate inside a living cell, stops reproducing and dies out.

However, certain viruses are known for their ability to survive in the human and cause persistent infection.

Dr M. Oldstone (1989), wrote this about persistent viral infections:

> Such viruses do not kill the cells, and do not elicit an effective immune response. These tactics enable the viruses to establish a long-term presence within cells, where they can have a subtle and persistent effect – by altering the specialized function of the cell, such as the production or secretion of a hormone. Such 'luxury functions' are not essential to the cell's survival, but may be vital to the health of the organism (e.g. a human). It is likely that immune, nervous and endocrine systems are primarily involved.

M.E. seems to be a persistent virus infection. Other diseases, such as diabetes, Parkinson's disease and schizophrenia, will probably turn out to be caused by persistent virus infections.

In M.E., a virus is probably affecting the special function of brain cells, and indeed many other organs of the body. Some endocrine functions may be affected, such as the pituitary gland, thyroid gland, the adrenal glands (which produce hormones of vital importance in the body's reaction to stress and infection – see page 114), or ovaries. The pancreas may be involved in some viral infections; this can lead to poor digestion of food, and also to diabetes. There is no part of the body which is never affected by a widespread, persistent virus infection.

A persistent virus would also continually stimulate some degree of immune response. This response is not great enough to destroy the virus, but has two main effects:

a) The constant production of cytokines, the chemical weapons made by white cells as part of an immune response. Interleukin 2 (a cytokine) when tried as treatment for cancer patients, caused such unpleasant symptoms – emotional lability, fatigue, muscle pains, and 'flu'-like feelings – that the trial was abandoned. Interferon had similar unpleasant effects when tested on patients with chronic liver infection.

b) The other effect of an abnormal ongoing immune response (to the persistent virus) is allergic reactions (see Chapter 14).

   Multiple allergies are common in M.E. – 'The patients' medical histories reveal one striking finding: a high frequency of atopic or allergic illness – up to 70 per cent' (Komaroff and Buchwald 1991).

The question is often asked: is someone with M.E. or CFS infectious to those around them? The viruses that may cause M.E. are carried by a large percentage of the population, in the throat, nose or in the gut, without causing any ill health. It does not seem that people with M.E. are any more likely to spread these common bugs about than the rest of the population is.

It is estimated that roughly one in four of M.E. patients has a close relative or work colleague with the illness. In the case of more than one member of a family being affected, there may be factors other than the virus to consider, such as an inherited predisposition to the illness. The infectiousness of M.E. and other chronic fatigue syndromes is not yet clearly understood. At the present time, some physicians in the USA recommend caution to patients – this includes advice to people with M.E. or CFS not to be blood donors.

So, assuming that a variety of viruses, and indeed other infections and even immunizations, trigger off M.E., what other factors are involved? Why is it that a number of people in a community can be infected with something – say an enterovirus, which seems the most likely virus where M.E. occurs in 'outbreaks' – but only a few develop the M.E. syndrome? And how can one explain the origin of typical M.E. in a person with no obvious infection at the onset? These patients, who report a gradual loss of health and onset of fatigue and end up with classical M.E. syndrome, present the greatest challenge for diagnosis and for understanding how their illness came about. It is likely that one of the main factors which determines whether you get M.E. is the efficiency of your immune system (see Chapter 4).

Muscle Studies

Dr L. Archard (1988) examined muscle biopsies from 96 patients with PVFS; using a special technique, he found enterovirus-specific RNA in 20 cases. It was not present in any of the healthy controls. The percentage positive for enterovirus may be an underestimate, because a biopsy specimen may not always include a sample of muscle affected by virus.

Prof. P. O. Behan and colleagues, Glasgow (1991) recently published important research. Using a new technique (Polymerase Chain Reaction) they identified enterovirus RNA in 53 per cent of the biopsies of 50 patients with typical features of post-viral fatigue syndrome. In 41 controls, enterovirus RNA was positive in 15 per cent (all positives were in patients undergoing surgery for cancer).

The enterovirus found by this PCR method was studied further by sequencing the molecules of its RNA.

This revealed that the virus was a possible variant of poliomyelitis and most closely resembled polio vaccine. Further studies have shown that this particular sequence resembled a cell protein *calsequestrin*, which is involved in calcium metabolism.

(Behan, 1991, British Medical Bulletin, p. 808)

These findings may be important in studying cell malfunction in M.E. Further research on this is going on at present.

Dr Archard (1990) published further work on enterovirus RNA which showed a mechanism that explains why enterovirus becomes persistent in a small minority of people:

Muscle biopsies from PVFS patients that were positive for enteroviral RNA were used. The production of virus RNA in these samples was compared with RNA production in cultured cells infected in the laboratory. The results showed that there is a defect in the way the enterovirus in the M.E.-affected muscles reproduces itself. The normal virus 'identification code' therefore may not be present, and the virus does not multiply. The immune system may not recognize the defective virus RNA, does not destroy it, nor produces an inflammatory response.

The same phenomenon is seen in dilated cardio-myopathy (a serious condition which may necessitate a heart transplant), a presumed progression from a viral myocarditis, and so may be a general mechanism of enteroviral persistence.

Mitochondrial Abnormalities

Dr D. Doyle (1991) described a study of 130 patients whose muscle biopsies were examined by electron microscopy. Mitochondria are tubular structures present in every cell nucleus. They are the cells' power stations, where energy is produced from a metabolic process using oxygen and glucose. Abnormalities were identified in functions, energy storage mechanisms, and the appearance of mitochondria. Samples were studied for presence of virus particles, and positivity for the virus correlated with electron microscopic abnormalities of mitochondria.

In another study (Behan et al., 1991), examination of muscle biopsies from 50 patients showed abnormalities of mitochondria in 80 per cent, and in none of the 50 controls.

It is tempting to speculate that a persistent virus might interfere with mitochondrial DNA, leading to muscle fatigue. Similar damage to the central nervous system might account for the psychiatric features, described in this syndrome and for the hypothalamic dysfunction which we have recently identified.

Electromyography (EMG)

Jamal and Hansen (1985, 1989) carried out single-fibre EMG on 40 patients. Abnormally high 'jitter values' (measurements of muscle fibre irritability) were recorded in 70 per cent of the patients.

In a further study, single-fibre EMG was carried out on 10 patients with PVFS. *All* the patients showed abnormal jitter values. Muscle fibre density was normal in each case.

A muscle membrane disorder, probably arising from defective myogenic enzymes, is the likely mechanism for the fatigue and the EMG abnormalities. This muscle membrane defect may be due to the effects of a persistent viral infection.

Muscle biopsies were carried out on these 10 patients. All showed some abnormal findings in their muscle fibres, and in the mitochondria of all patients, which suggested a problem with cell energy metabolism.

Four of these patients had nuclear magnetic resonance (NMR) studies carried out (see below): all had positive results.

All these findings confirm the organic nature of the disease.

Nuclear Magnetic Resonance (NMR)

Arnold, Radda and Bore (1984, 1985) have demonstrated *early excessive acidosis* (excess lactic acid in muscle tissue) in the exercised muscles of patients with post-viral fatigue syndrome, using Nuclear Magnetic Resonance (a method for assessing biochemical changes in tissues). Muscles of patients were tested during exercise, and excess lactic acid was produced abnormally early. The conclusion drawn was that there was a defect in the balance between the two kinds of energy production.

In M.E.-affected muscle there may be too much of the anaerobic energy pathway (which uses glucose) compared to the aerobic route (which uses oxygen), causing excess lactic acid production. This could account for the muscle pain and severe malaise after exercise that accompanies M.E.

Electron microscopy had already shown an increase in size and number of Type II muscle fibres, (Jamal, above) which are the muscle fibres that use the anaerobic pathway, releasing lactic acid.

Abnormal Protein Synthesis in M.E. Muscle

Prof. Peters (1991) examined muscle biopsies from M.E. patients for RNA, DNA, and protein content. There was a significant 17 per cent decrease in total RNA per cell. Further studies demonstrated a decrease in muscle protein synthesis in M.E. patients (Pacey, 1988). A lessened ability of muscle to repair itself might contribute to the rapid fatigability of M.E. muscles.

At Biolab in London, Drs S. Davies and J. Howard have developed a test of muscle function which uses fine heat sensors to record muscle activity – a *myothermogram*. In the muscles of M.E. patients, their recording of muscle activity is grossly abnormal. The contraction is normal, but the relaxation of muscle fibres is slow and jerky, and at rest the muscle shows continuing activity (Howard, 1989). There might be an imbalance of magnesium and calcium across muscle cell membranes associated with this abnormality.

In spite of all the foregoing evidence of abnormalities in muscles of people with M.E., several studies have demonstrated 'that chronic fatigue syndrome is not a muscle disease. Muscle function is not impaired' (Wood, Edwards et al., 1991). However, the flaws in these studies have been (a) to ignore the muscle findings, and (b) to use patients complaining of chronic fatigue (e.g. in one study the patients were taken from those attending a 'fatigue clinic'), which includes patients who do not have M.E./PVFS. It seems most likely that the abnormal muscle fatigability found in typical M.E. has causes both in the muscle cells and also in the central nervous system.

Fibromyalgia

Fibromyalgia is a chronic condition characterized by muscle pain, tender points ('fibrositis'), stiffness and sleep disturbances. It has therefore some clinical features in common with M.E. and with CFS. In a study of primary fibromyalgia, only 7 out of 33 patients diagnosed as having primary fibromyalgia fulfilled criteria for CFS (Wysenbeek, 1991). It is probable that some people diagnosed as having fibromyalgia may have M.E. However, fibromyalgia responds to exercise therapy, to local injections into tender points and to low-dose amitriptyline (a tricyclic antidepressant), which improves the sleep disorder. The sleep disturbance is a disorder of alpha EEG rhythm (part of a brain wave recorded during a sleep electro-encephalogram). Fibromyalgia symptoms may also be mediated by cytokines, as is true for CFS symptoms.

Chapter 4

What Causes M.E.?

II – Immunology, Red Cells
and Neuropsychiatry

In those patients whose M.E. came on gradually, with no precipitating viral infection, it is possible that they had some previous virus which remained dormant in the body, not causing any immune reaction. Then for some reason there was *something which damaged their immune system*, thus lowering the body's resistance, and the latent virus became active and triggered the M.E. syndrome.

Factors which may injure the immune response:

Viral infections – e.g. glandular fever, hepatitis

Acute stress – emotional shock, accident or assault

Prolonged unrelieved stress. There is a close relationship between emotions, the endocrine glands (hormones) and the immune system

Immunizations [this connection remains unproven, however]

Dietary deficiencies

Environmental injury – such as from pesticides, ionizing or electromagnetic radiation, chemical pollution

Bowel infestations – parasites (Amoeba, Guardia Lamblia), yeasts, bacteria. Intestinal parasites, particularly Guardia Lamblia, are suspected by some researchers to depress the immune system, and untreated intestinal Guardia could pave the way for developing M.E. later from an enterovirus. This may partly explain why there appears to be a high incidence of getting M.E. after a spell abroad. Diagnosis of Guardia Lamblia is difficult, and may involve a biopsy of the small intestine, or Guardia antibody in stool (Galland 1989, 1990).

The Immune System and M.E.

The picture of immunological abnormalities in M.E. is at present rather confused, because various studies have found a variety of abnormalities in different patient groups, sometimes with conflicting findings. So far there is no single test of immunological function that is consistently abnormal in 100 per cent of the cases. It can, however, be said that all the research results taken together do indicate that immune dysfunction occurs in M.E. syndrome.

These are some of the more significant studies:

Dr P.O. Behan (1985) and colleagues in Glasgow studied 50 patients with PVFS. The following immune abnormalities were found:

- Reduced function of lymphocytes to make protein
- Abnormal numbers and ratios of T-cells
- Circulating immune complexes were present in 25 per cent of the cases
- Autoantibodies (antibodies to a patient's own tissue) to various tissues were found in many patients

Dr Lloyd (1989) of Australia investigated 100 M.E. patients.

Immune abnormalities were:

- Reduced levels of IgG1 (Immunoglobulin G1) and IgG3 in 56 per cent of the patients. (This finding was confirmed by a later study).
- Reduction in numbers of total lymphocytes and T-cells. T-cell function (cell-mediated immunity) was reduced in 88 per cent of the patients, compared to 1 per cent of the healthy population.

  '. . . this provides the strongest reported evidence of disordered T-cell function in patients with CFS.'

- Increase of lymphocytes showing immune activation. 'Once activated these cells may continue to produce cytokines, which mediate the symptoms of CFS.'
- Levels of Interleukin 1 (Klimas, 1991), also of Interleukin 2 (Cheney, 1989) have been measured in CFS patients and found to be much higher than normal.

Klimas et al. (1990): In this study of 30 CFS patients, the most consistent abnormality was *low natural killer (NK) cell cytotoxicity* – virally infected cells were not being killed properly. The authors state that their results: '. . . suggest that CFS is a form of acquired immunodeficiency. This deficiency of cellular immune function was present in all the subjects that we studied.'

Komaroff and Buchwald (1991), in a review of all laboratory findings in CFS, comment on the inconsistency of immune abnormalities:

> In some studies, even those who meet the case definition of CFS may have been suffering from different illnesses in which fatigue is the common denominator. Tests are obtained at various points in the clinical course, a circumstance that makes it difficult to determine if abnormalities are transient or fluctuate over time.

That is, immunological findings may vary at different stages of the illness.

The authors summarized all the most consistent findings from all published immunology research:

- Depressed numbers and function of natural killer cells
- Low levels of circulating immune complexes
- Low levels of several autoantibodies, particularly antinuclear and antithyroid antibodies
- Altered levels of immunoglobulins
- Abnormalities in the number and function of lymphocytes

The most recent findings of abnormal immune function

in M.E. (Landay et al., *Lancet*, 1991) indicate that there is *immune activation*, the degree of which is directly related to the severity of disease. Specifically, the abnormalities were in subsets of T8 suppressor cells – further details are too complex to describe here.

Of the patients who were severely ill (capable of less than 25 per cent of normal daily activity), 85 per cent had one or more abnormal results; whereas of those patients who had largely recovered, only 10 per cent had abnormal results. The abnormal immunological markers were not found in healthy controls, nor in groups of patients with conditions such as depression, chronic fatigue alone, acute viral infections, and SLE (a chronic systemic illness).

Red Blood Cell and Cell Membrane Abnormalities

Dr Mukherjee (1987) and colleagues in Australia examined red blood cells from seven M.E. patients at the time of a clinical relapse. In four cases, some of the red cells showed an abnormal shape. Such abnormal red cells had previously only been seen in the blood of runners after a marathon. M.E. sufferers in relapse say 'I feel as though I have run a marathon' after minimal exertion. On retesting three weeks later, when the patients felt better, there were no abnormal red cells.

Dr Simpson (1989) of New Zealand looked at red blood cells from 102 patients with M.E., also from 52 healthy controls and 99 Multiple Sclerosis (MS) patients. Samples from M.E. cases had 'the highest incidence of cup forms and the lowest percentage of normal red cells'.

The significance of these research findings is the fact that red cells have to change shape slightly to pass through minute blood vessels (capillaries), which they can do if they have the normal bi-concave disc shape and a flexible outer coat. If some cells are deformed then these might not squeeze so easily through capillaries, resulting in reduced blood flow and oxygen supply to some tissues.

Dr Simpson (1991) found identical red cell abnormalities in blood from M.E. patients in California, Western Australia and the UK, associated with M.E. symptoms. Vitamin B_{12} injections led to improvement in well-being within 24 hours, and loss of symptoms was associated with reduced numbers of abnormal red cells in half the cases.

There are symptoms suggesting impaired blood flow in M.E.: areas of poor perfusion in the brain (see page 69), poor muscle performance during exercise, impairment of cognition and other intellectual functions (as after a stroke), and poor circulation in the hands and feet.

A possible explanation of abnormal red cells in M.E. came from Dr Wakefield (1989): Excessive cytokine production, e.g. interferon, due to persistent viral infection, can produce structural changes in cell membranes, this could account for some deformed red cells in patients in relapse.

In a study on 25 CFS patients (Kajid, 1991), all of whom had red cell membrane abnormalities, I.V. infusion of 15 gm ascorbic acid (vitamin C) led to significant return to normal of the red cells. Further studies are needed, yet this gives some rationale to the anecdotal reports from some patients of the benefit of high doses of infused vitamin C.

Magnesium in Cells

A study at Southampton (Cox et al., 1991) found low levels of magnesium in red blood cells of subjects with M.E., compared with healthy controls. A therapy trial of magnesium injections produced improved symptoms and stamina in 80 per cent of the M.E. patients, and raised their red cell magnesium levels to normal (see page 164).

The reason why intracellular magnesium appears to be low in M.E. is not clear, and the above study is being repeated.

Neurological Abnormalities in M.E. and CFS

Possibly the most crippling disability, especially in the long-term patient, is the loss of intellectual abilities, collectively known as 'cognitive dysfunction'. This is what causes many M.E. people, who in their thirties and forties are skilled professionals, to lose their jobs. Physical disablement is hard enough but can be coped with; many other people with physical disability can function intellectually and hold jobs, compute, create, and contribute some wage-earning activity to society.

When someone of normal or above-average intelligence finds that his or her memory, concentration, comprehension, even speech is disturbed by this disease, is it any surprise that he or she becomes depressed and anxious? As well as cognitive dysfunction, emotional disturbance is common with M.E.: depressive symptoms, acute anxiety, panic attacks, and sometimes euphoria and mania. This kind of emotional lability is also common in MS.

Depression and anxiety are such common symptoms of M.E. that some doctors attribute all the M.E. symptoms to untreated depression.

However, depressive symptoms commonly occur with any chronic illness. A depressed person 'suffers from lowering of mood, reduction of energy, and decrease in activity. Capacity for enjoyment, interest and concentration are impaired, and marked tiredness after minimum effort is common' (International Classification of Disease). But this is not a description of someone with M.E., who typically is well motivated, enjoys things he or she is capable of, and does not have sustained lowering of mood. Depressive symptoms, especially profuse weeping, are directly associated with exhaustion, fever and feeling very ill (perhaps as a result of from cytokine activity? – see page 54), and usually improve with rest.

> Diminished ability to think, concentrate or remember may be caused by an organic mental disorder, and are not useful symptoms for making a diagnosis of a major depressive episode in the medically ill. Since fatigue and loss of energy are so commonly caused by physical illness, these vegetative symptoms cannot be used to make a diagnosis of major depression.
>
> *(Cavanaugh, 1991)*

If you take a number of people with M.E. (not just 'chronic fatigue'), who have a condition causing a brain disturbance with disordered neurotransmitters, and excess cytokine production by activated white cells; an illness which makes many lose much of their lives – jobs, family, friends and sports; an illness with debilitating exhaustion, pain, and malaise – would you not expect those affected to show emotional disturbance some of the time?

If you modified these emotional symptoms, would you expect to cure the underlying disease?

There is also a relatively high incidence of depression in other diseases that affect the brain, including Alzheimer's, MS, Parkinson's disease and Huntingdon's disease (Schiffer, 1990).

In one survey of people with MS, it was estimated that 'the lifetime risk of depression is 40–50 per cent, and that cognitive deficits are present in 60–70 per cent [of the] patients' (Stenager, 1990).

In another study of MS, it was found that an increase in emotional disturbance coincided with an increase in disease activity (Dalos, 1983). About 80 per cent or more of MS patients suffer from severe, disabling fatigue; another similarity with M.E.

In some M.E. research studies there is not a strict enough case definition for patients, and probably much less than half of cases with 'chronic fatigue' have M.E. or post-viral fatigue syndrome. In one study, only 5 per cent of patients presenting with 'chronic fatigue' fulfilled the American case definition for the Chronic Fatigue Syndrome (Manu, 1991).

Neurological Research Findings in M.E. and CFS

There is now evidence that the cognitive dysfunction represents organic neuropathology – there is something wrong in the brain that can be seen or measured.

The following findings were presented at two meetings – at Los Angeles, February 1990, and at the M.E. Symposium at Cambridge, April 1990:

Dr Carolyn Warner, who specializes in MS, found neurological symptoms in many CFS cases, the most prominent being balance disturbance. On certain neurological tests patients lose balance and fall over, and more complicated tests of vestibular function are abnormal.

Dr Shiela Bastein, (Berkeley, CA) carried out a range of *neuropsychometric testing* on 175 people with CFS. These tests pick up different defects in cognitive function. She found definite abnormalities which, when put together, made an identifiable pattern of dysfunction unique to CFS.

Magnetic Resonance Imaging

(MRI – same as nuclear magnetic resonance) brain scans are done regularly on other patients with neurological diseases, and have been performed on many CFS patients of all age groups in the USA. The abnormalities on MRI scans indicate patches of inflammation in various areas of the white matter of the brain.

In the Lake Tahoe epidemic, 80 per cent of patients had brain MRI lesions. In California, endemic (isolated) cases also were 80 per cent positive (compared with 21 per cent positive in healthy controls). Non-specific MRI changes in brain scans increase with age; this causes scepticism about MRI findings in CFS patients. However, Dr Cheney looked at positive MRI scans in different age groups; in ill teenagers with CFS over 50 per cent had abnormal MRI scans – quite abnormal for this age group.

Northern Nevada Epidemic Data

Daugherty and colleagues carried out cognitive function testing on 20 CFS patients and 20 healthy controls, and found significant dysfunction in 19 of the 20 CFS patients. The most marked and frequent defects were in attention-concentration, problem solving, kinesthetic ability, and verbal memory.

MRI scans were done on 15 of these patients and 16 controls. There were abnormalities in *all* the CFS patient scans, but only one from the healthy control group. The striking distortion along with the abnormal results of MRI scans in these patients suggest a pathological process in the brain. *The pattern of focal and lateral impairments is more consistent with that of an atypical organic brain syndrome, than of anxiety and depression'* (Daugherty, 1991).

A comprehensive survey was carried out in the USA (Buchwald et al, 1992) in which 259 patients were studied, all of whom had an illness that started abruptly after a 'flu-like' episode. They all had features of disabling chronic fatigue and impaired cognition. Results of the study included:

- MRI brain scans showed scattered sub-cortical foci of inflammation in 78 per cent of the patients.
- A higher average ratio of CD4/CD8 T-cells than in healthy controls.
- Active replication of human herpes virus type 6 (HHV-6) in 70 per cent of patients (see page 52).

The authors comment that 'neurological symptoms, MRI findings, and lymphocyte studies suggest that the patients may have had a chronic, immunologically mediated inflammatory process of the central nervous system. The active replication of HHV-6 most likely represents reactivation of latent infection, perhaps due to immunologic dysfunction.'

SPECT Scan

This technique looks at blood perfusion of the brain. Professor Ismael Mena did a study of SPECT scans on CFS patients and on healthy controls. He found perfusion defects in 71 per cent of the CFS patients, mainly of the right temporal lobes. He did a further test in which CFS patients exercised on a bicycle. Their SPECT scans were repeated after vigorous exercise (when blood carbon dioxide had returned to normal), and there was a *decrease* in blood flow to the brain, mainly in the temporal and frontal lobes. The expected result would be an increase in cerebral perfusion after exercise (Mena, 1991, *CFIDS Chronicle*).

The SPECT scan abnormalities are especially interesting because they corresponded with the neuropsychometric data, which said that the temporal lobe was most likely to be affected – based on knowledge of various psychological functions of different areas of the brain cortex. This clinical and laboratory correlation makes a powerful argument for there being some abnormality of the brain in M.E./CFS.

Electro-Encephalo-Gram

Dr Jamal, of Glasgow (who did single-fibre EMGs, page 57) found EEG abnormalities in 85 per cent of 20 PVFS patients tested. These changes suggested a patchy disturbance of cerebral function.

Hypothalamic Function Studies

The control centre of many bodily functions – e.g. appetite, temperature, blood sugar, sleep pattern, sweating, mood, libido, body weight – is in the hypothalamus (part of the mid-brain). M.E. symptoms include upset of many of these functions, so research in the UK and USA has looked at hypothalamic function.

In Glasgow, studies have shown that patients with PVFS/M.E. have abnormal water balance – when a loading dose of water is taken, the hypothalamus does not regulate the hormone that tells the kidneys to conserve or flush it out, and patients tend to retain water. This might partly explain the erratic weight gain of such patients. Such water-retention also occurs in irritable bowel syndrome and premenstrual syndrome.

Further work, testing the hypothalamic response to a substance called *busiprone*, compared the response of PVFS patients to that of patients with primary depression. The PVFS patients showed a significant rise in the amount of the hormone *prolactin*, but the depressed group had no rise in prolactin. This prolactin response is a way of testing *5-hydroxytriptamine* (5HT, a chemical that affects mood) receptors in the hypothalamus (Behan, 1991, *British Medical Bulletin*).

Other recent research on the hypothalamus has shown evidence of a fault in the hypothalamus-pituitary-adrenal hormone regulating system. This fault appears to be a deficiency in *Corticotrophin Releasing Hormone* (CRH) from the hypothalamus. The end result in the patient is abnormally low levels of plasma cortisone in the evening, and reduced 24-hour urine excretion cortisol levels. This is a simplification of the published research paper, which is very complex (Demitrack et al., 1991).

However, the authors point out that 'glucocorticoid [a cortisone hormone] deficiency can result in immune abnormalities perhaps sufficient to contribute to the exacerbation of allergic responses and raised antibody titres to a variety of viruses that are seen in CFS patients.' Viral infections may affect hypothalamic CRH release by altering neurotransmitters (see page 124.) This recently published research may prove to have further implications for unravelling the complex symptoms of M.E.

Some young M.E. patients have been seen with Parkinsonism, which usually gets better in a year. Iceland researchers have also found a higher-than-expected incidence of Parkinson's disease among the now middle-aged people who were involved in the 1948 Iceland M.E. outbreak.

Most M.E. symptoms, including Parkinsonism, memory loss and the hypothalamic dysfunctions, could be explained by upset of the mid-brain functions – one could call it a 'mid-brain syndrome'.

Other Studies of Behaviour and Cognitive Functions

Hickie and others in Australia (1990) assessed 48 patients who fulfilled criteria for CFS, using a range of psychological interviews and tests, and compared data with that from 48 matched controls who had depression.

Of the CFS group, 80 per cent reported the following psychological symptoms:

Poor concentration – 52 per cent
Poor short-term memory – 27 per cent
Depression – 38 per cent

The pre-illness rate of major depression and all psychiatric disorders was no higher than that within the general community. In addition, the pattern of psychological symptoms was found to be significantly different to that of the depressed control group, and severe depression was rare.

The researchers concluded:

There is no evidence from our well-defined sample to support the hypothesis that CFS is a physical variant or expression of a depressive disorder. Instead, our study supports the hypothesis that the current psychological symptoms of CFS are a consequence of the disorder, rather than evidence of antecedent vulnerability.

In the UK, Prasher, Findlay and colleagues (1990) measured sensory-evoked and auditory event-related cognitive potentials in 37 patients diagnosed with M.E., and in 25 healthy controls. A *potential* here means measurement of an electrical change in the brain that results from a stimulus – a sound stimulus, or a peripheral nerve stimulus, or a visual one.

There were no abnormalities found in the pathways of sensation of vision, sound or from peripheral nerves. However, cognitive potentials that measured attention and efficiency of information processing (identifying two different sounds, and responding to them) were different in the patients. 'The abnormalities indicate attentional deficits in some patients and speed of information processing in others. The prolonged latencies observed in these patients have not been observed in patients with depression in many other studies.'

Andrew Smith (psychologist, University of Cardiff – ongoing research) uses tests of performance efficiency in patients with evidence of chronic viral infection (VP1 positive or abnormal muscle biopsy) and controls. The test results so far show that M.E. patients have:

• Impaired motor function
• Greater sensitivity to visual stimuli
• Slower ability to search for targets
• Increased distractibility
• Impaired short-term memory

These results suggest that behavioural measurements may help to distinguish between chronic enteroviral illness and depressive illness.

So, after all these studies looking at the illness from many different aspects, what is causing the M.E. syndrome?

a) There is a persistent virus infection in some cases.
b) Something has upset the immune response:
   A previous virus? A new virus? Environmental factors? Stress? Parasites?
c) Physical overexertion at the time of an infection may have an adverse effect (as with polio).
d) Probably some inherited predisposition
e) Continuing immune response produces excess circulating cytokines, which may be damaging cell membranes, impairing blood flow, and interfering with brain function.
f) Continuing psychological factors may be perpetuating the illness in some cases.

If you are confused after reading about some of the research into M.E., you are not alone! There is as yet no single expert who can explain exactly what causes M.E. and the mechanisms of all its distressing symptoms.

There may be some alarm and confusion arising from the publicity about HIV/AIDS and its causes, and a possible link with M.E. In M.E. there may be some abnormal immune response, *but this is quite different to the immune collapse seen in HIV/AIDS.*

Chapter 5

M.E. – The Diagnosis

At the time of writing this book, there is no test for M.E. which gives a clear *yes* or *no* in 100 per cent of suspected cases.

It has been suggested that, as there is no treatment and you just have to live with it, there is no point in going to your doctor if you suspect you may have M.E.

A recent TV programme in the UK set out to show that getting a diagnosis of M.E. had not helped those patients who had been selected to take part in the discussion. The arguments were not convincing; however the programme probably sowed seeds of doubt in the minds of many M.E. sufferers, who were on the brink of having their illness accepted by their GPs and families.

The point of diagnosis was brought home to me very forcibly, when, on the same day that this particularly unhelpful TV documentary was shown, I read a report of a young man who had just committed suicide. He had been ill for over a year with a 'chronic virus', had typical encephalitic symptoms of M.E., and muscle fatigue. His work performance had deteriorated so much that his employers gave him notice to quit. The loss of a job to someone who is struggling and ill, and is not recognized as such by employers – who should otherwise have discussed sick leave, can be the last and fatal straw.

So there are good reasons for you to seek a diagnosis if you think you may have M.E.:

You need to rule out other conditions, some of which may be treatable – you may *not* have M.E.
You need a diagnosis, in order to apply for time off work

or a change to part-time work, to apply for Social
Security benefits, home help, retirement pension, etc.

If you are at school, you need the diagnosis to allow you
to rest at home when ill, without your parents being
prosecuted for your non-attendance (yes, this does
happen to parents of children with M.E., hopefully
less now that the illness is better recognized).

You need to know if you have a genuine illness in order
to stay sane. To be told that your inability to stand up,
to work normally, to think or live a normal life is not
psychological is a wonderful relief, and may save some
from suicide.

Through knowing what is wrong, you can start to
reorganize your life, and come to terms with the
illness.

Getting a diagnosis is, for many, the starting point of
improvement. Battling on in ignorance of the problem
is a sure way to get worse.

You need all the support and understanding you can get.
It is hard for your doctor, family and friends to supply
this when they do not realize that you are really ill.

The more experience your doctor has of patients with
M.E., the better his or her ability to help you and other
sufferers.

Through getting a diagnosis, you can be put in touch
with others through patient organizations such as the
M.E. Association.

If you have *not* got M.E., you will be very glad to know
it. Other possible reasons for the symptoms and
fatigue can be discovered and dealt with.

With so much publicity about the illness in the past year,
a good number of people are going to their GPs to say
'Have I got M.E.?' when they may just be overtired or run
down through inappropriate lifestyle. This puts doctors
in a quandary, because M.E. is not a disease which is
taught in medical schools, or seen much in general
hospital wards; and if it is, it is called something else,

such as heart attack, abdominal pain, or nervous collapse of unknown cause.

The diagnosis is made on the basis of a patient's history, and lack of objective signs of other disease. There are sometimes abnormal signs on physical examination of the nervous system, and there are a number of laboratory tests which may help confirm the diagnosis (but even if the results of these prove normal, this does not rule out M.E.)

A list of symptoms typical of M.E. is given in Chapter 1. The cardinal symptom is *fatigue*, unrelieved by rest, and made worse by exercise.

When you go to your doctor, or to a specialist, do prepare some sort of history of your illness in writing, in advance. Write down:

• When you last felt well
• All infectious illnesses you have had, especially any that occurred around the time of the onset of your current symptoms
• Anything else that happened to you just before the onset
• If anyone in your family or work circle was ill at the same time, and if any of them developed symptoms of M.E.
• Your main symptoms at present
• Whether the symptoms have been constant or intermittent
• How your illness has affected your lifestyle – work, family life, income, social activities
• How much exercise you could take when you were well, and what you can do now without ill effects
• Anything that seems to make you better

This preparation will help the doctor, and save you from forgetting important information at the time of consultation – most M.E. patients have a bad memory which only gets worse when under a cross-examination! If possible, take along a relative or close friend who knows you very well, and who can add his or her observations about any changes in you since the illness, should your mind become a blank.

If your illness has begun shortly after a viral infection (sometimes up to 6 weeks later), and you have classical symptoms, then the diagnosis is fairly easy. It is much more difficult in the case of someone who has become unwell gradually, with no obvious precipitating infection. For these people, it is especially helpful to try and remember past infections or bouts of unwellness, which may be as seemingly trivial as a 24-hour tummy bug while abroad.

Your doctor should enquire about childhood illnesses, previous health, operations, and drugs taken (especially antibiotics). Also about the health of your parents and siblings, and a family history of allergies, undue infections, or M.E.-type illness.

A full physical examination should be carried out, including blood-pressure, examination of heart, lungs and abdomen, a search for enlarged glands, and tests of neurological function and muscle power.

There is rarely extreme muscle wasting, but there may be some loss of muscle bulk, especially in the thighs. This is usually symmetrical, unless one limb is worse affected.

Neurological tests may show brisk tendon reflexes, but the *plantar* response is usually normal (the big toe curls down when the sole of the foot is lightly scratched), and there is no *clonus* (jerky contraction of a muscle when suddenly stretched). Two tests which are sometimes abnormal are the vibration sense and the Romberg test (sense of balance with eyes closed).

Simple tests of muscle power may be normal. However, if muscles are exercised – such as the patient squeezing a rubber ball for one minute, or being sent to climb 40 stairs (if able), the muscles used will be found to be weak, the weakness lasting several hours or several days.

There is almost invariably muscle tenderness. Careful fingertip feeling of the thigh or upper back (trapezius) muscles usually reveals points of great tenderness.

A key factor in arriving at a diagnosis of M.E. is the exclusion of other diseases which might be causing fatigue. Briefly, these would include chronic infections, endocrine diseases, nervous system disorders, cancer, muscle diseases, auto-immune disorders, and primary psychiatric illnesses.

There are a number of blood tests which should be carried out, as well as urine testing, and then possibly more specialized investigations for M.E. or to exclude other conditions. Muscle biopsies, electromyograms, and the enterovirus test (VP1) are not routine tests, but may be used as part of some research programme.

Nevertheless, ultimately the diagnosis rests on a careful history, and exclusion of other conditions. Once a doctor has seen a patient with M.E., the symptom picture is not forgotten. It is fair to say that many doctors are unsure about recognizing the illness, or even believing in it, until they know one of their patients, one of their family or a colleague who develops it; this experience usually dispels any scepticism, and any other patients in the practice who have M.E. will benefit thereafter.

Details of the differential diagnosis, and a routine of investigations (one of which is carried out by a consultant physician in Bristol who is interested in M.E.) are given in Appendix B; this may be of interest to doctors and other health workers.

Chapter 6

Plan of Management

As you probably know, you cannot go to your doctor and come away with a prescription for a drug which will cure M.E. Take comfort from knowing that most M.E. sufferers get somewhat better in time. There is strong evidence to show that those who rest early in the illness have a better chance of recovery.

Present estimates are that if you have a diagnosis of M.E. and you have been ill for less than a year, you will have about a 70 per cent chance of recovery within 5 years. Of course this means that 30 per cent will still have M.E. after 5 years. However, this is an illness which usually has ups and downs, and if you can learn to manage your life with M.E. then you are unlikely to stay at your worst all the time. It is natural to remember only the worst times, the days when you feel absolutely awful, but think also of the days when there has been an improvement in energy, and the feeling that life may still be good.

There are three broad categories that describe the course of the illness:

1. Those who gradually get better, then stay better.
2. Those who have remissions and relapses (the remissions may last for several years), but never seem to shake the disease off permanently.
3. A small number of unfortunate people in whom there is no remission, and who remain ill for years.

Keeping a Diary

I have found it helpful, when going through a bad time, to refer back to a good day and to imagine myself in that happier state again. For this reason I think that keeping some sort of diary is useful. Much has been said about the value of writing down all the bad symptoms as they occur, and what you have eaten, drunk, and done – especially looking at exercise. In this way you may see a pattern developing that shows what things cause a relapse in you.

But it is just as important to commit to the diary the *good* days, the experiences that have given you pleasure or made you laugh, anything that has caused an improvement. As most M.E. sufferers have poor memories, a diary can be useful to refer to before going to see your doctor, and to look at the results of any therapies you have tried. It is best to try to develop a routine of scribbling something every morning or evening. Even a weekly diary is useful.

However, there are some people for whom the idea of monitoring their illness suggests that they might be a hypochondriac. This is understandable: the British in particular do not think it is 'quite the done thing' to take too much interest in one's aches and pains. But if you take an interest in the good times as well as the bad, then optimism may balance the hypochondriasis.

Another good reason for keeping a record over a period of months is that it is hard to remember exactly how you were six months ago, and while there may be ups and downs the general trend is more likely to be one of very gradual improvement, which will only become obvious when you refer back to the diary. The decision to keep a diary is an individual one. If you are too ill to write, perhaps your carer can keep some sort of a record for you.

Helping Yourself

What has happened in a person with M.E. is a lessening of the body's defence system which deals with viral infection.

Factors Known to Decrease the Immune System Function

Virus infections can cause a reduction in numbers and function of lymphocytes.

Stress – especially if protracted. This includes physical stress caused by, for example, exposure to cold or exhaustion, and mental or emotional stress such as is caused by bereavement, overworry, divorce.

Nutritional deficiencies

Refined carbohydrates – i.e. glucose, sucrose and fructose – reduce available vitamin C and impair white cell function.

Certain drugs – such as steroids, anticancer drugs, the contraceptive pill, possibly some antibiotics (by upsetting the natural balance of friendly bacteria in the body), and immunosuppressants used after transplants.

Exposure to chemicals – including smoking, which depletes the body of vitamin C.

Recent research has shown a definite link between psychological stress and immune functioning (*Lancet*, June 1987). What seems to be relevant is not the amount of stress one is exposed to, but how one handles it; thus someone who remains depressed for a long time after a bereavement or serious family illness has a greater chance of becoming ill him- or herself. So the observation by many M.E. sufferers that they thought they had undue stress for a period before developing M.E. is logical. If severe stress had led to their immune system not working so efficiently, then their bodies would not be able to deal with a viral infection properly.

The aim of any plan of management should be to encourage the body to mobilize its own healing forces. We have an amazing capacity for healing and repair of damage in our bodies; unfortunately, for all sorts of reasons this healing force is often suppressed, as explained above. Anything that will allow the immune system to become stronger and to overcome the persistence of viruses in our cells, should be valuable for an M.E. sufferer.

A person with M.E. has little energy. Therefore it is vital that none is wasted on unnecessary activity. This includes physical activity, worry and anxiety, and the energy required for digesting the wrong foods, and for getting rid of chemicals or drugs.

If the immune system is having to deal with other foreign agents, or allergic reactions, it will not have enough resources to deal effectively with a continuing viral infection.

Your state of health results from the balance between things that decrease your healing energy, and those things that promote recovery.

Negative Factors	*Positive Factors*
Too much exercise	Physical rest
Lack of sleep	Sleep
Worry	Freedom from anxiety
Mental strain	Mental rest
Work stress	Relaxation
Sadness, bereavement	Calmness
Loneliness	Love and friendship
Cold and damp	Warmth
Hunger	Joy, laughter
Wrong food	Good, nourishing food
Sudden shocks	Fresh air and sunshine
Surgery	Lack of chemical pollution
Most drugs	Avoiding infection
Anaesthetics	Patience and optimism

Infections
Poisons (alcohol,
chemicals, smoking,
pollution, etc.)

If you look at these lists , you can see that all the positive factors are the sort of things we try to give our children and those we love. When you are ill, you need to spoil yourself a bit, to give yourself those good and natural things you would wish for a loved one. It is unrealistic to expect others to provide them all, though if you have love and support from others it is a tremendous help; but you *can* organize quite a lot of positive forces for yourself.

In planning a campaign for living with M.E., it is best to do it in stages, and have an order of priority. There is not yet enough evidence that the following suggestions will be helpful in every case, however reducing exertion and resting seem to be essential for all sufferers. Other lines of management have *all helped some people*. The advice offered is not aimed at achieving a total cure, but rather to lessen the severity, encourage more remissions, and help you to live more comfortably with the condition.

It is not much use spending money and time on various treatments and at the same time continuing to live on an 'overdraft of energy', so *rest* is the first thing to organize.

Things to Do to Help You Cope with M.E.

• Organize your lifestyle to allow for more rest
• Stop unnecessary exercise
• Learn to relax – e.g. meditation
• Accept your limitations
• Improve your nutrition, avoid low blood-sugar levels
• Keep warm at all times
• Take nutritional supplements, especially vitamin C

- Avoid chemical pollution
- Deal with candida infection if present
- Treat any allergies
- Get more fresh air and daylight
- Learn to handle depression, with treatment if necessary
- Develop positive thinking and serenity (of course this is difficult on bad days!)
- Do not be shy about asking for help
- Apply for things to make life easier (social services, walking aids, etc.)
- Contact other sufferers for support if you feel isolated, such as joining a local M.E. group
- Do not compare yourself with other people who have your illness; some will be more ill, some less, they all have ups and downs like you.

In learning to live with M.E., half the battle is won if you can accept that you just *cannot* live at the same pace as you did before you became ill. To do this you need to realize that your worth is not measured by achievements in terms of being busy, earning money, athleticism or even being particularly good at anything.

Remember, you will probably improve.

The following chapters will talk about these things in more detail.

Of all these suggestions, *physical and mental rest* and *good nutrition* are the most important.

Chapter 7

Rest and Sleep

A person with M.E. is like a car battery that cannot hold its charge. The battery can be connected to charging leads overnight, and in the morning it appears to be full of energy, but after very little use the lights go dim, the engine won't turn over, and the only solution is to recharge it. Rest is all about recharging your battery.

The metabolic machinery in a M.E. sufferer has gone wrong. Energy is taken into the body via food, and oxygen from the air, but the transformation of these substances into useful energy is inefficient. The power station in each cell (called mitochondria) has a spanner in the works in the shape of a piece of virus protein. The cells which most obviously show up this defect are those of the muscle and brain.

When you use muscles, a by-product of the energy reaction is lactic acid, a build up of which causes pain. This pain and stiffness normally goes away in a day or two in a healthy person. But the M.E.-affected muscle accumulates lactic acid after relatively little work, and also takes far longer to get rid of it and recover.

If you start to feel exhausted, mentally or physically, there is little point in pushing yourself on, as the stage of complete collapse will soon arrive. Many sufferers find out by experience that more can be achieved in a day by doing only a little at a time, and having frequent rests, than by pushing on to the limit and then having to have a long rest. The problem in managing exercise and rest is that by the time you feel exhausted, you may have passed the stage at which a short rest will recharge you, and it may take several days of rest to recover. If you stop before this point, recovery may only take a few hours.

Establishing a Routine

A daily routine, in which you can do things in a rhythm of activity and rest, worked out to suit *you*, is recommended. During a period of severe illness or relapse your daily activity may be merely several trips to the bathroom and perhaps a short time spent in a chair by the window.

It is helpful to think of your available energy as resembling your available cash – as a bank balance. Lots of rest builds up your bank balance of energy. Each morning you will have a certain level of energy to use before you go into the red. If you have almost depleted the account the previous day, you may start out with the impression that you have plenty of energy in the bank, but will quickly find that you were only just in the black, and go overdrawn early in the day.

Each day you (and only you) have to decide how best to spend your energy quota. Usually it has to be spent on 'basic housekeeping' – eating, dressing, excretion, maybe shopping or cooking. If you want to do something exciting or frivolous – in my case to attend for two hours' practice with my choral group – you allow for this by taking extra rest before or all day, and do not complain if the next day you are overdrawn!

However unwell you may be, you are likely to have a daily pattern to your energy – some wake up feeling reasonably human, but steadily run down as the day progresses. These people need to plan to do essential things early in the day, to make most efficient use of what energy there is. Many others wake up (if they have slept) feeling they would rather be dead, and by later on may improve. For them, things to be done should be arranged for later in the day. It is worth telling friends and colleagues when to call, and when not to bother you. This saves the awkwardness of being incoherent on the phone to someone you'd otherwise love to talk to.

If you are well enough to think of working full- or part-time, and this can be arranged, it obviously pays to try and organize your working hours to suit your best time of day. This will be less stressful on both you and your colleagues, as well as more efficient.

Having said all this, I do realize that there are sufferers who find no pattern to their levels of energy at all. However, if you keep a diary of ups and downs and of what you have been doing, then some sort of pattern may well emerge.

Learning to Rest

The more you rest early on in the illness or during a relapse, the quicker you will improve.

Resting, and the giving up of a lot of activities which were part of a busy life, requires discipline. In the past decade we have been bombarded with exhortations to take exercise in order to be healthy. The streets and parks are full of joggers, friends always seem to be planning 'activity' holidays such as ski-ing, sailing, or walking. We are conditioned now to think that if you sit all day in a chair you will become ill or get 'furred up' arteries, and for a healthy person this may be true. Success tends to be measured by visible achievement; keeping busy is reckoned to be good for one's morale; people who live 18-hour days and appear to be healthy and successful are much admired.

If you have M.E. you must *unlearn* all these conditionings. You will have to learn to be a Mary instead of a Martha, an observer and listener instead of a doer or talker!

Do try and think of the giving-up of activities as something *positive* to do, rather than negative and 'giving in' to M.E. Rest should be regarded as positive, constructive treatment rather than just as 'doing nothing'.

In restructuring your life, you will find that you have to 'spring clean' your priorities, and in fact some aspects of life become much simpler, because there will be fewer choices you have to make. For example: if you do not have the energy (or money) to go shopping for clothes, you will not have to face those exhausting hours and indecision in clothes shops, and as you do not go out so much, the clothes you have will be adequate.

Contentment can come from simple things; the secret of coping is to lower your sights, to *move the goal posts a lot nearer*. Then you will be able to score an achievement more often, with a great deal less effort. Then a walk to the local shop can be as exciting as a weekend walking in the country. A beautiful sunset can be as pleasurable (and cheaper) as a trip to the cinema.

It is important to accept the things you cannot do, and to make the most of what remains. Also to remain optimistic about the future, and to continue to believe that gradual improvement is possible. During the time that you are ill, you must not be too proud to ask for help where needed. Most people like to give and to help, and are waiting to be asked. There may be a forgotten relative who could help, or a lonely neighbour who would be happy to do some shopping or look after the children sometimes. It is worth asking your doctor, or the Citizen's Advice Bureau, about what sorts of help are available, until you are better.

Do remember that your health is more precious than money, and that none of us is indispensable at work. The office, patients, or workshop, will all be there when you get better. So will the possibility of doing other things, even if you lose your job through illness. Many unemployed people, without M.E. or CFS, also have to learn to cope without a job in the present economic decline. Obviously each M.E. or CFS person must decide how best to reorganize life. It is usually a question of sorting out priorities, and your top priority has to be to get better.

I have a scarlet sweatshirt with a motif that reads: *Non Omnia Possumus Omnes.* This is Latin for 'It is not possible to do everything.' I have to remind myself continually of this. It's a good motto for anyone with diminished energy, struggling to get through the day.

Gentle Exercise

In the early stages of the illness, as much rest as possible should be obtained. At this time one should not try to do anything more than the bare minimum. Some people worry about loss of muscle bulk and power from lack of use. In fact the shrinking of muscles is not as great as one would expect, nothing like the wasting that happens in paralytic diseases such as polio. However, if you are ill enough to be spending all day in bed, and if this is likely to be for weeks, then it is essential to do some very simple and non-strenuous movements each day. Every joint should be moved through its full range, to avoid the development of contractures or a stiff joint; and gentle stretching of the whole body should be attempted, as is done by a cat on waking. This can be done yourself, or very gently by a carer.

Suggested Movements

- Shoulders: lift each arm slowly forwards, up beside your ears, back as far as possible, and down.
- Elbows: straighten each arm completely, then bend it so that your hand touches your shoulder.
- Wrists: keeping your forearm still, make a circle with your fingertips, rotating your wrists.
- Fingers: curl them up, then straighten them, then spread them wide apart.
- Neck: starting with your chin on your chest, make a slow circle in both directions, so that your neck bends forwards, then sideways, then backwards, to the other

side, then forward again.

- Hips: lying prone or on one side, take your leg backwards, return to starting place, then take it sideways. These movements need not be great, but are important to prevent your hips becoming stiff and bent.
- Knees: gently straighten your legs from time to time, so that your knees are not bent continually.
- Ankles: rotate each foot, first clockwise and then anticlockwise.
- Back: lying prone for a while each day should extend your back. Back tension can be eased a bit by bringing your knees to (or near) your chin, then releasing them again.

The object of these movements is to prevent stiffness or deformity of joints. Most patients will be doing enough each day for this immobility not to become a problem – having a bath, drying off after the bath, putting on clothes, walking round the house. Even if you have to spend much of the day in or on the bed, you should change out of your nightclothes into something else which is warm and comfortable during the day.

There is a fine margin between lying in bed and doing absolutely nothing, losing muscle bulk and tone, and maintaining enough mobility to keep your body supple and maintain muscle tone, while still having enough rest. The other reason for moving around is to keep some circulation going to your extremities, which tend to get cold anyway.

It is also important to aim for some increased activity after the initial period of illness, that is – when the sore throat, fever, muscle spasms and sweating have diminished. Fear of exercise-induced symptoms may prevent a sufferer from ever trying anything new. Do remember that mild symptoms of muscle aching, dizziness and fatigue are inevitable when starting even gentle activity after bed rest that has lasted more than a few weeks. Mild symptoms will settle quickly, and should not be a reason to collapse back in bed. Even if you inadvertently overdo things during a slow increase in activity and have M.E. fatigue and relapse, this will not harm you, and with rest these symptoms will settle down again.

Sleep

This is the best form of rest. During sleep the rate of repair of body tissues is greatest. Animals and children sleep the clock round when they are ill. Many M.E. patients complain that they seem to need too much sleep, but you should allow yourself to sleep as much as you can, it will do nothing but good. If you don't sleep well, you cannot get well.

Unfortunately, a good night's sleep is hard to achieve for many people with M.E. or CFS. All sorts of things conspire to prevent it: muscle or joint pains, oversensitivity to noise, muscle twitching, palpitations, sweating, nightmares, breathing difficulties, panic attacks, and a racing brain that just will not switch off even though you are exhausted.

So, if you have chances to sleep in the day, take them. If you expect to spend some time awake during the night, have some distraction at hand, such as a radio or an undemanding book, and also something to eat. Try not to fret about being awake; this wastes energy and stops you relaxing.

Suggestions for helping you to sleep:

- Go to bed before you become exhausted and allow yourself time to relax, e.g. with quiet radio or an easy book.
- Make sure your bed is comfortable. If your muscles are very sore, put a quilt, duvet or sleeping bag under the lower sheet. If you are spending a lot of time in bed, consider investing in a washable sheepskin to lie on.

The mattress should be fairly soft but not sagging. I have found a good quality latex foam (non-inflammable) mattress better than a sprung one, and also better insulated (hence warmer) – but this is just my personal preference.

- Make sure you are *warm* enough. Chilliness increases muscle tension. An electric blanket is a boon for aching limbs even in summer (but make sure you switch it off before you go to sleep).

- Essential oils, especially Lavender, in the bath or gently massaged into the limbs, really do help. If you can get someone else to do this for you, even better. You can find out more about the properties of various oils by consulting an aromatherapist or reading a book on the subject. It is important to use only oils that are calming or relaxing; those that are stimulating should be avoided. Lavender seems to be good for most M.E. people: it relaxes and calms muscles and balances body energies.

- Avoid exciting or distressing TV, radio, or books in the evening. If one is emotionally fragile, one can weep through the night about some tragedy seen on the news.

- Do not go to sleep hungry, for you will wake up at 2 or 4 a.m. feeling awful – hence the wisdom of having a snack nearby just in case.

- Make sure your bedroom is properly ventilated; there does not need to be a gale from the window, but an airtight, stuffy room does not provide enough oxygen, and may increase indoor air pollution.

- Ear plugs are a boon if you are extra noise-sensitive; they muffle street noises, courting cats, ticking clocks and snoring spouses. The best are the soft wax ones, which soften in the ear, fit snugly, and are non-irritating. They are also useful on a noisy train or bus, or in any situation when noise is an irritation. In summer they can be at hand when sitting in the garden, to put in if a neighbour's lawn mower starts up.

- Avoid having lots of electric cables passing across or near the head of your bed, and if possible switch things off at the plug before sleeping, except for a bedside light. Electromagnetic energy fields may not affect healthy people, but M.E. sufferers seem to be extra-sensitive to them, and sleep disturbance may be one of the effects.
- There are various herbal teas available which are mildly sedative and non-addictive, e.g. Chamomile, and special night-time mixtures. Avoid tea or coffee after 4 p.m. If milk does not disagree with you, then an old-fashioned warm milky drink at bedtime is worth trying. Heated milk contains calcium and natural tryptophan (an amino acid, a component of protein), which are both sedative, and the calories help prevent night starvation.

Sleeping pills are in theory best avoided, as they can lead to dependence on them. However, if nothing else works, and you are suffering night after night and feeling exhausted in the morning, then taking a mild sedative for a few weeks does no harm. Once you start to feel a bit better you may be able to do without them, or take them on the odd night only. A short-acting one like Temazepam (5 to 10 mg) should give six to seven hours of sleep and not make you groggy in the morning.

Some anti-depressants are sedative, and some more than others. For intractable sleep disturbance, which is such a common symptom of M.E., a low dose of an antidepressant such as amitriptyline (10–20 mg to start with) at night can be useful. Sleep disturbance is a common feature of a condition which resembles M.E. called fibromyalgia, and good results have been obtained in a trial of a very low dose tricyclic antidepressant in this condition (amitriptyline 10–20 mg at night). A test of such treatment for sleep disturbance in M.E. is awaited. Some cannot tolerate side-effects of antidepressants, but side-effects are less common when the drug is taken in a very low dose.

In the early stages of the illness or during a relapse, the symptoms that result from doing too much develop within a few hours or the next day. With recovery, the time lapse between overdoing and getting the symptoms (that prove that you shouldn't have attempted overdoing) gets longer, and it becomes more difficult to relate cause and effect. The muscle pain, weakness, sweating or feeling awful may not happen until two days following the imprudent exertion. If you are still keeping a diary it may show you what has caused the relapse. With recovery, the length of time needed to come out of a relapse should get shorter, maybe one week of rest instead of three months; maybe one day instead of a week.

Beware – during the time of gradual recovery, it is very tempting, when feeling so wonderfully well (comparatively), to forget you still have M.E. and to do something stupid like running for a bus or shifting furniture. I know some people whose sudden extreme exertion has put them back to bed for months.

Mental Rest

There are various levels of physical rest, ranging from weeks in bed to an hour sitting in a chair. But it is very important to have mental and emotional rest as well. Most of us have a constant chatter of thoughts whizzing around in our brain while we are awake.

If you are used to a busy job (and this includes running a home), then quite likely when you were well you were able to have three levels of thought going on at once.

For example: The most conscious level is holding a conversation; the middle level is composing a shopping list; the deep level is worrying away about some unsolvable problem such as your child's bad school progress.

Sound familiar?

With M.E. this sort of mental acrobatics is nearly impossible, and leads to confusion and brain fatigue. The short-term memory goes, so by the time you reach the third item on your shopping list you have forgotten the first two. You struggle wearily upstairs to get something, only to forget what it is you wanted when you get there.

The brain intellectual functions that are affected by whatever it is – cytokines or virus X – that's interfering with the normal messages passing between brain cells are: short-term memory, ability to do simple arithmetic, abstract reasoning, concentration, and interpreting information.

Brain fatigue is as real as muscle fatigue. It is no good trying to force your brain to cope. Many of the circuits and terminals in the computer in your head are out of order; some days more circuits will function than others. Computer experts have coined the term 'virus trouble' to describe some mysterious malfunctions in computer systems – I wonder if these boffins have experience of M.E.?

People with this kind of brain disorder learn to write everything down – and end up searching in exasperation for shopping lists, telephone numbers, etc. I have found no solution yet to the mystery of vanishing lists, nor vanishing clothes, key rings, or tin openers. All this is apparently caused by *not* being able to make memories properly, so a visual imprint of car keys sitting where you put them simply is not filed in the brain. Then, if you have also lost the ability to make associations between things and places, it is not surprising to find the keys in the middle drawer and your pile of clean underwear on the hall table!

The frustration experienced at losing things, or forgetting what they're called, is very wasteful of mental energy, and for previously mentally agile patients this can be harder to bear than the physical fatigue.

If the confusion comes on quickly during the day, it may signal the need for some food and/or a rest. The best thing to do if a sudden fog comes over you is to stop whatever you are trying to do, have something to eat if it is three hours or more since your last meal, and have a little doze. Many M.E. people manage to stay in a job by negotiating flexible hours and arranging for somewhere to rest if their energy suddenly runs out.

The same principle – of stopping before you reach complete exhaustion – applies to brain fatigue as well as muscle tiredness. For months I simply could not cook a meal at 6 p.m., and I struggled and cried over the difficulty of co-ordinating my brain and hands with the cooker, even to boil potatoes. Then I started the routine of a snack at 5 p.m., followed by another rest, which also improved the edibility of the food.

There are various techniques for learning mental rest, including meditation, hypnotherapy, or listening to relaxation tapes (see Chapter 9).

Adjusting

Do remember that when you have M.E., all your functions need to be adjusted so as not to waste precious energy. You need to work out new patterns of behaviour, and to do this effectively you need to listen to what your body and mind are telling you.

One way of looking at the illness is to see it as our body going on strike, and demanding new terms and conditions of employment. Most people with M.E. are by nature highly energetic, and other people tend to look to them for support and enthusiasm. M.E. seems to thrive on these patterns of behaviour.

(From an article written by an M.E. patient)

It may be that a lot of M.E. people will not make any real progress until certain patterns of living have been unlearned, and other more energy-conserving behaviour has been learned.

Getting M.E., or any fatigue syndrome, is a clear message that something is wrong. The illness has forced you to come to a full stop, and fighting what is happening is the worst thing you can do. So give in gracefully, stop fighting yourself and the world; rest, and rest some more, and let the world go by for a time. Unless you do this, the disease is likely to take an even deeper hold.

Case History

The following story is told by a lady who has had M.E. for 22 years, and illustrates the importance of rest:

Miss W. T., now aged 71, retired

'I was first ill in 1970, when I was 49. It was thought at the time to be a virus infection – there were a number of funny viruses around at the time.

'There were years of relapse and recovery, years of weak legs, years of apparent good health, and a steady decline starting in the winter of 1982–83, until the summer of 1985 (when I started to adapt to my life instead of trying to fight it). Since then the only relapses have been when I was in hospital for tests and forced to exercise for physiotherapy or testing. For the last two years I have been able to live at barely 50 per cent of normal life.

'My symptoms are: muscle weakness, which causes me problems with standing, walking, carrying. Fatigue. Pain and jumpy legs at night, sensitivity to noise, inability to concentrate for long; sleep disturbance – my brain may race and I cannot relax, or I may go to sleep, then wake feeling disturbed by a bad dream. I'm also very sensitive to changes of temperature, and sometimes my words get muddled.

'When I am very tired, I am clumsy and irritable, and my face goes a nasty yellow-grey colour.

'I had many medical tests done: for glandular fever (result:

normal), for an underactive thyroid – normal, a gland biopsy, repeated tensilon tests – normal, a muscle biopsy – a slight abnormality, repeated electromyograms – mostly normal, one slightly abnormal, a skull X-ray and CT scan – normal, a psychological interview – normal!

'I got almost as many diagnoses as I had tests: 1970, 1972, 1976 – ''virus infections''; 1984 – ''nothing wrong with you''; 1985 – damage to nerve in muscle, cause unknown; 1986 – nothing neurologically wrong – advised to see a psychiatrist! Later in 1986 – damage to muscle, could be due to earlier virus? 1987 – M.E. (after 17 years!)

'I worked out that the muscle weakness dated from the old virus infection (1970), but doctors would not listen to me. In 1986 I heard a radio talk about M.E., and it sounded like me. I sent off to the M.E. Association for more information, and I became more convinced. Later I found a consultant who is familiar with M.E., who confirmed the diagnosis, without doing further tests.

'In the light of my experience during the last four years, I cannot stress too much the need for rest, and for adopting a lifestyle in keeping with one's limitations. Right from getting the initial virus, I wanted to keep going, and was encouraged to be as active as possible as soon as possible. Since my troubles really started in about 1984, doctors have continually told me to keep going, and even when I was diagnosed as having irreparable damage and told by my GP to adapt my lifestyle and keep within my limits, the neurologist was still assuring me that I must *not* rest, I must keep as active as ever possible.

'It was during the time that I was fighting against the weakness, and dragging myself about in an effort to keep going, that my condition deteriorated so fast and so permanently. As soon as I modified my life and listened to what my body was saying and kept within my limits, whatever anyone said, it was amazing how the deterioration slowed down and almost stopped.

'The M.E. Association theory is that rest in the initial stages can be a big factor in recovery. I never had that rest. And now,

I cannot help wondering whether, if I had been advised to rest even in 1984, instead of being instructed to keep going, I might not have the permanent damage which has now occurred.'

Chapter 8

Exercise

How I wish that something as simple as gradually increased daily exercise could cure M.E. Exercise is an emotive word in M.E. circles, and the advice generally given by experienced M.E. people is: *don't do it*.

However, a lot may depend on what one means by exercise. At one extreme there is punishing exercise such as running and squash, in which a fit person pushes him- or herself to the limits of endurance and uses anaerobic metabolism. There is no evidence that jogging prolongs life, while it certainly wears out joints and running shoes. Heart attacks do happen to apparently fit young-to-middle-aged people during squash or running sprees (including the American man, Jim Fixx, who popularized jogging!). *Doing vigorous exercise while recovering from any viral infection can be dangerous*, as the heart muscle may be affected by any virus. I do not recollect any centenarian interviewed on radio or TV, when asked 'to what do you attribute your long life', ever mentioning jogging – more usually a gentle lifestyle, with a daily trip to the local pub!

The other extreme is the exercise involved in getting out of bed and putting on clothes, which may cause exhaustion in someone acutely ill with M.E. What may be more relevant is movement and activity, rather than exertional exercise. Suitable exercise for anyone convalescing from chronic illness includes walking, gentle swimming, yoga – and singing.

Why singing? It uses the muscles of the chest, throat and diaphragm. It is creative, expressive, increases oxygen intake and improves circulation; it is good for the spirit; if done with others as a group activity it is fun and sociable. If you sing while sitting, you do not use your leg muscles, which when affected limit nearly all activities that involve walking and standing. You may be surprised at my including singing as exercise, but it is an alternative to painting, writing poetry or making baskets, when more strenuous activities have to be abandoned. You don't even have to purchase the musical instrument.

Every town, and many villages, have amateur choirs and church choirs, which welcome enthusiasm as much as talent. Making music transcends all the differences in age, income, social class and state of health that may exist among participants. There have been times in the last two years when a weekly trip out to sing, even when unwell, has kept me sane. No one minds that I bring cushions and sit all the time.

Graduated Exercise and Cognitive Therapy

An alternative explanation of long-term disability in chronic fatigue syndromes has been developed by some British psychiatrists (Butler et al., 1991):

> Looking specifically at CFS, it is plausible that an initial infective trigger may begin a cycle in which attributional and cognitive factors fuel avoidant behaviour. The initial symptoms, in particular fatigue and myalgia, engender a state of 'learned helplessness' . . . and may trigger or exacerbate the mood disorder that is found in many patients. Avoidant behaviour sustains symptoms, by decreasing activity tolerance and increasing sensitivity to any stimulation, as does associated mood disorder. Re-exposure to activity causes more symptoms and more fear. The result is a vicious circle of symptoms, avoidance, fatigue, demoralization and depression, and the clinical picture of CFS.

This theory about M.E./CFS does not accord with the experience of most M.E. sufferers.

The treatment proposed by this group of doctors therefore consists of:

a) Treatment of depression (if present) with antidepressants
b) Gradual planned increase in activities that the patient feels comfortable with, including exercise
c) Cognitive therapy to help the patient break the association between activity and symptoms. 'If I feel ill today, it is because I did too much yesterday' (the logic learned from bitter experience by chronic M.E. patients) is changed to 'If I feel ill today, it is because I have been too inactive yesterday'!

A treatment trial of cognitive therapy and graded activity was carried out in a group of sufferers from chronic fatigue (Butler, 1990). Some of these conditions were self-diagnosed, some diagnosed as CFS by specialists – and the average length of illness was five years. 50 people were offered treatment: 32 accepted, and 27 completed the course, which lasted 4–6 weeks. The results were:

23 out of 27 who completed treatment felt better
Of those who fulfilled the criteria for suffering major depression, and who took a course of Prothiaden (a tricyclic antidepressant), 60 per cent improved.

There was an association between lack of improvement/worsening and patients who believed that their symptoms were due to physical disease, as well as those who had positive VP1 (enterovirus in blood). Could I suggest that these 'treatment-resistant' patients actually had M.E. proper?

The overall result was that 74 per cent felt improved after 4–6 weeks. After a further three months, however, this figure had dropped to 65 per cent. It would be interesting to see how many of these people had a *sustained* improvement after a year at the increased level of activity, and how many had relapsed on exposure to a further viral infection, or other stress.

This approach to treatment does appear to benefit some people with chronic fatigue. However, I do wonder how many of those who accepted the treatment had M.E., how many fulfilled criteria for chronic fatigue syndrome, and how many had fatigue from untreated depression or other causes. I find it significant that having a positive VP1 test made a subject less likely to improve with this treatment. Probably those people had a persistent enteroviral infection, causing the 'therapy-resistant' disorder in their muscle metabolism.

Before I ever heard of 'cognitive behaviour therapy', I believed that one simple way to differentiate between someone with chronic fatigue due to psychological causes, and someone with muscle fatigue caused by M.E., was an exercise test such as the following:

The Bull-in-a-Field Test

Place the subject in a field. Introduce a fierce bull into the field, and shut the gate behind him. The subject provokes the bull (using a cruelty-free scientifically tested stimulus, of course). The activity and symptoms of the subject are monitored for 24 hours.

The subject with 'neurosis fatigue' will be seen to run briskly across the field, and get over the gate; the next day he will feel less depressed, as a result of the surge of adrenaline and endorphins associated with the hard exercise.

The subject with M.E. fatigue will be seen to walk or stagger or maybe run (if his condition is not too advanced) across the field and collapse by the gate; if alive and not mauled by the bull, the next day his symptoms of muscle exhaustion and pain will be much worse, he will complain of feeling ill and 'fluey', and he may be depressed and weeping.

This test has not yet been accepted for authentic medical diagnosis, nor scientifically tested!

Of course, the unnecessary avoidance of *all* exercise, and continuing prolonged bed rest beyond the initial acute stage of M.E. and other post-viral fatigue conditions, *can* lead to problems such as deconditioning of the heart, lungs and muscles, psychological problems, and maybe a belief that one is becoming a permanent invalid. Total lack of use does lead to muscle weakness and muscle wasting. Lying flat for too long causes poor blood-pressure control when getting up, and therefore dizziness. Initial attempts of exercise after a period of bed rest will probably result in weakness, unsteadiness, and muscle aching in unused muscles.

But too much exercise for an individual M.E. patient leads to symptoms of relapse. So what is the best middle course for someone with M.E. to follow?

Dr D. Ho-Yen, consultant microbiologist at Inverness, who has studied a large number of post-viral fatigue patients, has pointed out that there are various sub-groups of patients. Which sub-group they fall into may affect how quickly they recover, and how they respond to exercise (Ho-Yen 1990). It is evident when looking at any form of management of this illness, that each patient must be assessed individually; what helps one may be useless for another.

There is no doubt that complete rest in the first weeks or months of a post-viral illness is helpful. Pushing oneself to exhaustion while convalescing from *any* infection delays recovery, and may lead to chronic disability if it is an enteroviral infection. It is during the chronic stage that a *gentle* increase of daily activity may be advisable.

Dr Ho-Yen has written:

Patients' experiences do not show that avoidance of exercise is maladaptive. It is proposed that the recently ill often try to exercise to fitness, whereas the chronically ill have learned to avoid exercise. Recovery is more likely to be achieved if patients learn about their illness and do not exhaust their available energy.

Available energy is the key to planning how much to do. As you (hopefully) gradually improve, you will slowly increase your bank balance of energy. It takes a long time, and one day of over-optimistic exertion may push your energy balance back into overdraft for weeks.

One of the things that told me clearly that I was ill, before I had even heard of M.E., was my *changed* response to any exercise. Previously, if I felt tired and low in spirits, I used to go for a brisk walk, or dig the garden, say at weekends after a busy working week. This exercise would always cheer me up, give me a good night's sleep, and refresh me for the next week. After developing M.E. I found that even the most gentle exercise would completely shatter me, and led to my feeling ill, hurting all over and crying for no reason. This dramatic alteration in the response to what is considered healthy exercise, is the most classic symptom of M.E., and should distinguish it from other fatigue syndromes.

Another thing not sufficiently appreciated by many doctors, is the difference between the fatigue felt by a normal person after a game of tennis or a 12-mile walk, and that felt by someone with M.E. after minor exercise: The former is described as 'healthy tiredness', refreshes the mind, improves the appetite and leads to a good night's sleep. The muscles may ache, but are relieved by a hot bath and sleep. This sort of healthy post-exercise fatigue is known to be good for many cases of depression, and is aptly described in Rudyard Kipling's 'How the Camel got his Hump' (one of his *Just So* stories).

But the post-exercise fatigue typical of M.E. is *quite different*, and needs to be experienced to be understood – it is not just tiredness, it is feeling horribly ill, collapsed, as though poisoned, with visible muscle twitchings, intense pains in the muscles and maybe in the joints; nausea, sweating, insomnia and nightmares; maybe an elevated temperature and recurring sore throat and tender, enlarged glands. This fatigue (an understatement) is *not* relieved by a good night's sleep.

How Much Exercise is Safe?

After trying out some new activity or exercise, see if the activity produces a gentle, healthy tiredness, or if it leads to M.E. fatigue. However, even if mild tiredness is produced, the patient needs to be very cautious and slow about increasing the activity. Unfortunately there is no easy predictor of whether an activity is going to harm you.

As an illustration – with apologies for using anecdotal evidence – a few months ago I had a bad experience with physiotherapy, prescribed to help treat arthritis in my hands. I managed two sessions of trying to comply with the physiotherapist's instructions – pulling on a coiled spring of 30 lb tension, to 'improve my upper arm strength'. I am still baffled by the logic of this exercise. The day after the second session, my body rebelled and went into a M.E. relapse that lasted over a week, with all the symptoms mentioned above.

When well enough, I went back and tried to explain that weight-training made me ill, and asked for gentle hand movements. But I was told by the expert physiotherapist that 'we all know now that M.E. is psychological; what *you* need is to stop lying around, and do more exercise.' I was astounded by this ignorance, and hurt; I had spent the previous hour struggling to do Christmas shopping in preparation for two guests over the holiday. I caution all M.E. *patients against physiotherapy unless the therapist understands the nature of M.E. muscle function.*

Feeling too ill to argue with her, I decided not to expose myself to further stress, so did not go back. However, I did find that *very gentle swimming* in a local, heated pool, was acceptable to my body, provided I did not exceed four slow lengths, and did not go on days when my muscles hurt.

Unfortunately, there is usually no warning bell to tell you when you have done enough, whether you are swimming, walking, gardening, or doing yoga in your bedroom. By the time you start to feel tired or your legs hurt, you have exceeded the safe limit. The only thing to do is to try something; if it proves to be harmful, rest until recovered, then try it again but *only do half as much*. Learn to read your body carefully to distinguish between symptoms of healthy tiredness, and those that threaten a relapse. Another important way to achieve more activity is to stick to a daily schedule of rest and activities, and then to vary the activities during the day, so as not to exhaust different muscle groups, or your brain.

For example, if during one day you aim to do a total of two hours' paper work, plus half an hour of gentle walking (maybe an ambitious day for some people), plus four hours of bed rest, it will work out better if these activities are split up and rotated – such as 10 minutes' walk, one hour rest, ½ hour paperwork, etc. Much more is achieved this way. Some M.E. people manage to return to a job by negotiating staggered hours of work, with rest during the day.

There seems to be a difference in response to exercise among M.E. patients in the early stages of the illness or in relapse, and among those in relative remission who may be able to cope with exercise better than when they were first ill. I do realize that much of this chapter may be useless for severely affected chronic M.E. people; I am aware of their plight.

You will find that *your body is the best judge* of how much, how often and what type of exercise to do. If you have features of fever, muscle twitchings, spasms, and muscle weakness, your body is telling you its muscles need rest. After a period of rest (not necessarily total bed rest), if the muscles stop complaining and you feel less ill, you may be able to start some gentle daily exercise. If you get some warning symptoms back after the experimental exercise, it was probably too much. The secret is to stop *before* you start to feel tired.

If you gradually increase the amount you can do and get away with, you may reach a limit beyond which you just cannot go, without a relapse – no matter how motivated you are. This limit must be determined by you and *your body*, not by a well-meaning physiotherapist, psychiatrist, or friend. The limit will vary; it may be quite high during a period of remission, but may be drastically reduced following some adverse factor, such as catching a cold, exposure to chemicals, or physical or emotional stress.

The Heart and Exercise Capacity in M.E.

There are cardiac abnormalities in the acute phase of most viral infections, which largely disappear after six weeks. A study of heart function, at rest and with exercise, in CFS was carried out by Canadian researchers (Montague, 1989):

> On graded exercise testing, 20 of 32 healthy subjects achieved target heart rates, compared to only 4 of 31 patients . . . Patients with CFS have normal resting cardiac function, but markedly shortened exercise capacity, slow acceleration of heart rate, and fatigue of exercising muscles long before peak rate is achieved. The data are compatible with latent viral effects on cardiac pacemaker cells, or their autonomic control, and skeletal muscle tissues.

The authors noted that the patients were strongly motivated to exercise, and to gain further insight into their symptoms.

Belfast doctors (Riley, 1990) investigated aerobic work capacity in patients with CFS. 13 patients were compared with 13 healthy controls and with 7 people with irritable bowel syndrome. The CFS group had a reduced exercise capacity, a lower peak oxygen consumption, higher heart rate at submaximal levels of exertion, and higher blood lactic acid levels during final stages of exertion. There were normal carbon dioxide end tidal concentrations, meaning the CFS group did not hyperventilate (page 117). The authors concluded that reduced exercise capacity could be due to unfitness, but similar findings occur with muscle damage.

These two studies demonstrate that differing results produce conflicting opinions about causes of poor exercise and heart function in M.E. and CFS people. It would be interesting to repeat these studies on people with proven enterovirus-caused M.E. (as opposed to more generalized chronic fatigue syndrome.)

As stated in Chapter 3, there seems to be involvement of the heart in about 30 per cent of the cases of enteroviral M.E. In a letter 'Myalgic encephalomyelitis: post-viral fatigue and the heart', Dr N.R. Grist (1989) described myocarditis in mice infected by Coxsackie virus, and the similar mechanisms in Coxsackie myocarditis and cardiomyopathy in humans:

It seems likely that similar immunological and metabolic mechanisms in M.E. may also result from chronic infection, providing the organic basis of the post-viral fatigue syndrome . . . a condition with severe fatigability and recuperation through rest. The heart muscle does not rest, except terminally. Does 'post-viral dilated cardiomyopathy'[1] represent the result of post-viral fatigue syndrome of the unresting heart?

The point of quoting these medical writings is to remind you that too much, or the wrong sort of, exercise could damage the heart in a proportion of people with M.E. Any symptoms of chest pains, shortness of breath, or palpitations that occur during any exercise should be reported to your doctor, and investigated.

However, do not be too frightened by this; the risk of heart attack is far greater for joggers without M.E., than for M.E. people taking gentle, sensible exercise!

1. This is a serious, uncommon condition, a rare complication of Coxsackie infection, diagnosed as a separate entity from M.E.

Yoga

Yoga is beneficial for circulation and breathing, and seems to improve blood flow to the extremities and hence oxygenation of tissues.

However, yoga is only suitable for M.E. sufferers who are recovering, and the inverted postures which place strain on the neck must be avoided, as must any posture which needs prolonged muscle tension to be maintained. Your yoga teacher should be told you have M.E., and you should not push yourself in any way. The most useful aspect of yoga, the breathing and calmness, can be carried on at home, sat in a chair, and can be learned from a teach-yourself book.

T'ai Chi Chu'an

T'ai Chi is a very ancient, gentle, martial art, performed as a series of traditional movements that are intended to unite body and mind. It was developed many centuries ago, and is widely practised in China, Japan, and other countries round the world, for health, meditation, and enjoyment.

You may be surprised to read that a martial art is described in a self-help book for M.E. sufferers! But the movements in T'ai Chi are very gentle and flowing, more like dance; no force or sudden muscular effort is used at all. It can be learned by people of any age, weak or strong. Each muscle is very gently changing between use and relaxation; there is improvement of muscle tone, of circulation of the blood and lymphatics, there is gentle movement of all joints, and the slow turning of the body massages internal organs. It is good for maintaining muscle tone. There is calming of mind and body, and deep regular breathing.

There is on record that a T'ai Chi master, a Mr Liang, learned the art in middle age, after many operations and prolonged illness. He not only confounded doctors who had predicted his imminent death, but was still practising it at the age of 77.

There will be M.E. patients who are not well enough to learn T'ai Chi, because it is performed standing up, taking slow steps and moving the arms. It is recommended for people who are getting better or who are in remission, especially those whose muscle weakness or pain is not so severe. Once learned, T'ai Chi can be performed at home as well as in a class. Even doing a few movements for a few minutes between spells of lying down can be beneficial.

To summarize what has been said in these last two chapters, the *Self-Care Manual for patients with CFS* (Lappmed and Cheney, Feb. 1991) advises (and this includes M.E., although their advice about exercise and cycling may not be appropriate to all chronic sufferers):

'Rest is best' . . . most patients report that rest is the best therapy. You must restructure your life so that it is possible to stop what you are doing when your body says 'stop'.

Most patients report that restructuring their life is the most difficult task, but is ultimately a rewarding lesson that many enjoy sharing with others.

Adjust your daily schedule to accommodate your body rhythm. Follow a fixed schedule of retiring and arising at the same time each day.

Each day you are given a finite amount of daily energy. An inner sense of trial and error will tell you how much energy you have each day, and when you must stop.

You will feel your best by pushing almost to the limit of your daily energy allowance. At the least get up, bathe and dress each morning. Don't regularly exceed your daily energy allowance or you will risk relapse.

Laying down and resting during the day can earn you extra energy towards your daily limit; mental stress and emotional strain sap energy and lower your daily energy allowance.

Save your energy for important things. Hire others to do housework. Get a cordless telephone.

Daily exercise of some kind is essential to prevent deconditioning. On the other hand, never exercise so much as to exceed your daily energy limit or risk relapse. If able, embark on a gentle walking programme. Begin with just a minute or two each day, then try five, then seven, and so on. You may be able to try swimming or cycling later . . . progress gradually. Some exercise each day may actually give you more energy for the next day. *The trick is in knowing the limit of what is therapeutic as compared with what is harmful.*

Suggested Further Reading
Dr Darrel Ho-Yen, *Better Recovery from Viral Illness* (Dodona Books, The Old Schoolhouse, Kirkhill, Inverness 1VJ 7TE, 1987).

Chapter 9

Stress

The word 'stress' is quite fashionable nowadays, and is blamed for much ill health. But what is stress?

It is comfortable to think that stress is an outside event which happens to us – a car crash, floods and earthquakes. With this point of view we can believe that we have no control over how much stress we receive. We can say: 'Life has treated me badly, that is why I have become ill'. Or 'There are too many demands on me, I am exhausted – I have to strive so hard at work.' These are the attitudes of people who see themselves as victims.

Just as fever is not caused by germs, but by the body's reaction to infection, so stress itself need not cause ill health; it is the *reaction* to stress that determines if one is badly affected.

Stress means anything which disturbs the equilibrium of mind or body. The tendency of the living person is towards stability, whether of body temperature, blood sugar, or the emotions. So 'stress' has a broader definition than that of a difficult job or a demanding family. Extreme heat or cold, hunger, trauma, infection, exhaustion, or fear can all be stressors.

Dr Hans Selye, Professor of Experimental Medicine and Surgery at the University of Montreal, has studied the effects of stress on living things since the 1930s. He was the first to show that the adrenal gland cortex produces cortisone in response to any disturbance to the body. Selye performed careful experiments on rats, using exposure to severe cold as the stress. He observed three stages in the animals' response to repeated exposure to cold:

1. Stage one – a shock response to the first exposure to the stress, followed by a reaction, and then recovery.
2. Stage two – on repeated exposure the animals appeared to adapt and become resistant to the cold. In this stage, the adrenal glands enlarged, in response to a stimulus from the pituitary gland (located below the brain). The changes in the animals to counteract the stress became more permanent. The rats appeared to be coping.
3. Stage three – exhaustion. The rats gradually failed to thrive; in those that died, post-mortem investigations showed that the adrenal glands were shrunken and had ceased functioning.

Selye called these events the 'general adaptation syndrome'. These stages are similar in humans:

1. The first exposure to stress produces an outpouring of cortisone and of adrenaline, to prepare the body for 'fight or flight' – the initial arousal state. If the stress passes, this reaction settles, and the body returns to its status quo.
2. Repeated stressing leads to a stage of adaptation, and the arousal changes become more or less permanent. The person may appear to adapt, but general health declines. There are chronic symptoms such as migraine, asthma, rashes, high blood-pressure, heart problems, mental symptoms, and poor blood-sugar control. The body cannot remain constantly trying to adapt to stress without permanent damage.
3. In stage three there is a breakdown in the adaptation. The result is collapse and exhaustion. This may take the form of a heart attack, nervous breakdown, or perhaps a major illness such as cancer. The breakdown may occur following an apparently minor stress, which acts as the last straw.

The second stage of the general adaptation syndrome is the one in which most GPs see their patients, with a whole range of chronic non-life-threatening illnesses. At this stage, if the stress is removed, recovery can take place.

In M.E., the viral infection which appears to trigger it off may have been the 'last straw' for a chronically stressed system. Not all patients have been stressed before developing M.E., but the stress may not have been obvious – intensive athletic training can injure the immune system, yet the subject would have believed him- or herself to have been supremely fit! Maybe this is why many M.E. sufferers are those who were very physically active pre-illness.

But maybe the chronic stress was not emotional, nor overwork, perhaps it was exhaustion brought on by raising small children – or a major accident, or surgery, just before exposure to a common virus.

There are many stressors, but what is essential, if you reach the stage of adaptive exhaustion and become seriously ill, is to accept where you are, to stop struggling to adapt, and to allow your adrenal glands and immune system to recover.

Having M.E. is of course a continuing new stress. The patient is fighting to get back to work, to get a diagnosis, to cope with daily functions such as maintaining enough income to eat, to look after a family while ill, etc. Some cope better than others with M.E.-induced stress; some have emotional support and help, and helpful doctors. Others may live alone, or be accused of malingering by their GP and family. Practical support is the first major way to reduce stress. Other ways are: relaxation, learning to breathe properly, meditation, and counselling to gain insight into the reality of becoming ill, and the possibility of getting better.

The symptoms of M.E. appear to be greatly influenced by both mental and physical stress. Although the illness is triggered in most cases by a viral infection, which then becomes persistent, there is also a psychological dimension to M.E. and CFS. *All* illness has a psychological dimension.

Research into causes and treatment of M.E. can be hindered by the artificial division of disease into 'physical' and 'psychological'. (David et al., 1988). The mind and the body operate as one unit. A structural disorder in the brain can manifest in psychiatric symptoms – such as can be experienced after a mild stroke. A hidden psychological disorder can manifest as physical symptoms (e.g. abdominal pain); this is called 'somatization' in psychiatry. It is fashionable and acceptable nowadays to attribute ill health to stress. But in Northern European cultures it is not socially acceptable to attribute physical symptoms to mental illness.

So management of M.E. requires not only physical rest but also mental and emotional rest, and sometimes the treatment of mental as well as physical symptoms.

In M.E., there seems to be increased sensitivity to stress. The heart rate is raised, with accompanying palpitations, out of proportion to the stimulus of anxiety or minimal physical effort; the breathing is often disordered, with feelings of breathlessness, or of a weight on the chest; and nightmares, sleep disturbance and panic states are common. M.E. patients are constantly exhausted, sweat profusely, have unstable blood-sugar levels; their peripheral circulation is often poor, and their body thermostats don't work. They are oversensitive to noises, smells, touch, and pain, and are emotionally unstable.

All these symptoms can reflect an overactive sympathetic nervous system (a part of the nervous system controlled by the hypothalamus). In a study, Levine and others (1990) found average plasma noradrenaline levels – both when lying down and standing – were higher in 20 CFS patients when compared to normal controls. The authors suggest that patients with CFS have a dysregulated adrenergic system, a theory that could unify the diverse symptoms of the illness. The hormone noradrenaline, released in response to a 'fight or flight' situation, causes rapid heartbeat, palpitations, flushing, and sweating. These symptoms may respond to self-relaxation techniques such as meditation, autogenic training, self-hypnosis, etc.

The Hyperventilation Theory of CFS

Dr Rosen and others (1990) studied 100 patients referred to them with diagnosis of CFS. Measurements of end tidal (after breathing out fully) carbon dioxide levels were measured at rest, after a period of overbreathing, and after a 'think test' during which subjects were asked to recall stressful events. The results were compared with those of healthy controls. The authors claim that the results showed 'chronic habitual hyperventilation', testing positive in 93 per cent of CFS patients. Suggested treatment for this would be: Training in breathing techniques and relaxation; counselling, and education about the mechanisms of one's symptoms.

These results have *not* been duplicated in a further study on overbreathing.

A common symptom in M.E., during a relapse, is the feeling of 'not getting enough breath', commonly waking up the sufferer from sleep. Could it be that the disturbance of the mid brain and hypothalamus referred to by Professor Behan (page 69), affects some central controls for breathing? If the brain senses a shortage of oxygen, it stimulates deeper and more rapid breathing, which washes out carbon dioxide from the blood. Therefore 'chronic overbreathing,' as diagnosed by Rosen et al., could be yet another complication of M.E. in some patients, rather than its cause.

Dr P. Nixon, cardiologist at Charing Cross Hospital and one of the authors of the above hyperventilation study, has pioneered work on stress reduction and correct breathing for patients with high blood-pressure and heart disease. Looking at M.E. patients, he thought that their overbreathing 'was a symptom of fear or panic, that can be experienced by people who demand a lot of themselves and fall short in their achievements'.

Looking at these two new theories about M.E. and CFS – the hyperventilation one (above) and the 'inactivity' theory, proposed by Dr Wellesley and others (page 101), they rather contradict one another. The hyperventilation theory suggests rest, relaxation and improved sleep as treatment. The psychiatrists suggest that M.E. symptoms are perpetuated by inactivity and *too much* rest, and advocate increasing levels of activity as part of therapy.

Both these theories probably apply to some people complaining of chronic fatigue, but *not* to the causes, symptoms and long-term disablement of people with virally induced M.E.

Meditation

Meditation is a technique for getting very high-quality mental rest; but it is not only the mind that is quiet. Transcendental meditation, for example, produces a state of profound physiological rest of the body, at the same time as increasing mental alertness. Some people may be put off meditation because they have wrong ideas about it.

Popular Misconceptions about Meditation

Meditation is thought to require effort in order to control the mind, and thus to be difficult and mentally taxing.

It is thought to be appropriate only for a particular lifestyle – that of mystics and religious people who withdraw from the world – or that you have to join a sect or convert to a new religion.

Most people do not know about any of the bodily benefits of meditation; they think it is only for spiritual growth.

How Can Meditation Help M.E. Sufferers?

The effects of meditation have been extensively studied on subjects during transcendental meditation. There are different techniques of meditating, as well as other ways of learning deep relaxation e.g. self-hypnosis, or listening to relaxation tapes.

The physiological changes during meditation indicate a state of quietness of the sympathetic nervous system, i.e. the opposite of the 'fight or flight' arousal state:

- The heart rate is decreased, the blood-pressure lowered, and breathing is slower.
- Oxygen consumption by the whole body is reduced.
- Blood flow to tissues increases, leading to better removal of the metabolism's waste products and a lower level of lactic acid in the blood.
- Long-term meditation is found to decrease a person's resting cortisol levels, even when he or she is not meditating. This reduction of adrenal gland activity is the opposite of Selye's stress response, and must be beneficial for M.E.
- Regular practice of TM increases stability of the autonomic nervous system.
- There are demonstrated electro-encephalo-gram (EEG) changes during TM, indicating more ordered brain function.
- Sensitivity to noise is reduced, and there is improved temperature control.
- Gum inflammation was found to improve after TM – this may indicate a beneficial effect on the immune system, although this has not been researched.

Relaxation Techniques

There are classes for learning relaxation, and there are a great many relaxation tapes available. They range from simple instructions for physical relaxation to guided imagery (also known as 'visualization'). The patient who is too ill (or poor) to attend classes will gain a lot of benefit from obtaining a relaxation tape and listening to it regularly at home.

Suggested Further Reading

O. Carl and Stephanie Simonton and James L. Creighton, *Getting Well Again* (Bantam Books, 1986).

(This book is written mainly for cancer patients, but is valid for everyone suffering from a chronic illness.)

Leon Chaitow, *Your Complete Stress-proofing Programme* (Thorsons, 1985).

Chapter 10

Depression

There can be few people with M.E. who have not travelled down into the dark valley at some time during their illness. Depression is a very common symptom in M.E. and CFS, and only those who have experienced deep depression can really sympathize with others so afflicted.

There is a difference between depression and unhappiness/sadness. The latter is usually the result of bereavement, difficult circumstances, or perhaps the inability to adapt to a situation.

If someone grieves for a deceased loved one, their sadness is normal; but if the sadness continues for a long time after one would expect the grief to have settled, it may turn into depression.

Depression as an illness affects most bodily functions. The sleep pattern is usually disturbed, with early morning waking, and one's mood lowest at the beginning of the day, improving later. A depressed person may be cold and slow-moving, the appetite is poor, there is lack of motivation, and an inability to experience pleasure in anything – the symptom called 'anhedonia'.

However, with M.E., depressive symptoms are not constant, and may be present for a few days or a few hours only. As with MS, depression in M.E. usually correlates with disease activity, most commonly associated with general relapse, worsened by overexertion, and improving with rest. This is the converse to a depressive disorder with psychological origin (see page 103 – the bull-in-the-field test), where exertion improves one's mood.

People with M.E. suffering from *emotional lability* may experience black despair, non-stop weeping, and suicidal feelings for a few days, then wake up one morning feeling fine. Or they may be irrationally happy, laughing and excited (maybe over nothing more than waking up without pain) one day – this euphoria leads to delusions of ability and lots of activity such as housework, extra socializing and missing the afternoon rest . . . and what happens the next day? They crash with a bump into the state of weeping and exhaustion. This up-and-down emotional behaviour is not the same as a state of depression; it is more typical of organic brain disorder.

The best way to lessen the highs and lows is to live within a daily routine of rest and activity, so your energy is used wisely, as advised in chapters 7 and 8.

Another source of depression in M.E. is the natural grief reaction to the losses – of the former active self, of jobs, friends, sporting activities, maybe of a spouse. This loss is not unlike that of someone who retires or is made redundant after many active years in a fulfilling job. There is inevitably a sense of not being needed; the world carries on very well without you, a world in which we are judged by what we are seen to do and achieve.

This secondary depression is common to all chronic disabling conditions, especially when the future is uncertain, and is bound up with anxiety and fear about the future. And part of the reaction to finding yourself ill with M.E. is, naturally, anger. Anger, if kept inside and not expressed, turns into depression, with loss of self-esteem. Of course you are angry at getting M.E., and at such a very inconvenient time, when there is so much you were planning to do. Because one is flattened, inactive, and maybe inarticulate, the anger is overlooked and very often suppressed.

Expressing anger in a constructive way is often used as part of psychotherapy for all sorts of mental problems; however, if you are flat on your back and saving your energy to do essential things you will not feel like hitting pillows or shouting to vent your rage. Some people are angry with themselves, if they are led to believe that they have developed M.E. because of bad living or past mistakes. You would be surprised to know how many people feel guilty about being ill. The belief that sickness may be some sort of retribution brought on oneself is common, though not openly admitted.

If you have M.E. and depression, the loss of self-esteem is unfortunately reinforced by the loss of ability to work or function normally. Talking about these fears and grief with a trained psychologist or counsellor can help an ill M.E. person to come to terms with things.

However, sometimes there may be a more sustained period of severe depression, when short-term remedies do not help. The patient may be in a black despair for days or weeks, unable to see a way out of it, and while in this state has no chance of improving energy levels or other symptoms. There is commonly a feeling of isolation, that one is cut off from other people and from experiencing any contact with beautiful things. An unhappy person may be moved to tears by beautiful music or a glorious sunset. A really depressed person will hear or see such things and feel absolutely nothing except perhaps despair because his or her contact with them is gone.

With this sort of depression there is often lack of motivation, insight, or judgement. The general purposelessness of life is seen in contrast to the apparent industry and contentment of other people.

The really frightening thing about severe depression is that you hate being in that blackness but cannot climb out of it. Well-meaning friends suggest that you snap out of it, or read a good book, or think of the world's starving children. But when in this state, you often cannot read, listen to the radio, or speak on the phone.

Why is Depression so Common in M.E.?

There are a number of reasons why depression can afflict M.E. sufferers:

- All virus infections cause some degree of depression.
- Cytokines are the chemicals which help to limit a virus infection. When interferon (a cytokine) was used to treat patients for another virus, the side-effects complained of were fatigue, muscle aches, and depression. Therefore, many M.E. symptoms may be caused by continued production of interferon in the body as a response to a persistent virus.
- If the brain is affected in M.E., then quite a lot of neurological functions are interfered with. Transmission of impulses between nerve cells takes place via chemical messengers called *neuro-transmitters*. (Antidepressant drugs change the balance of these chemicals, and so influence mood – see page 130.)
- The brain's chemical reactions need various amino-acids (derived from proteins), vitamins, and enzymes in order to work. A lack of any of these amino acids or of enzymes leads to a deficiency of one or more neuro-transmitters, and this can greatly affect mood. Therefore, nutritional deficiencies that are caused by a poor diet, poor digestion or malabsorption may contribute to depression.

  If a person with M.E. has recurrent diarrhoea and poor food absorption, this will increase the risk of depression because of lack of amino acids and B vitamins. (Depression is an early symptom in cases of starvation, and beri-beri – vitamin B_1 deficiency).

No one has invented a way of doing a biopsy on the living brain. So, unlike muscle fibres, which can be biopsied and looked at with an electron microscope, brain cells affected by a virus retain their secrets, and we don't understand exactly what is going wrong. However, some of the brain tissues of people with M.E. who have committed suicide have been found to contain enterovirus (see page 50).

Depression should be seen as yet another nasty symptom of M.E., rather than as something to do with the personality of the patient. Many M.E. sufferers are people with no previous history of depression, and their behaviour can change alarmingly with M.E. Uncontrollable tears, terrible, black depression, despair, panic, suicidal thoughts – all these can be felt by someone previously regarded as well-adjusted and in control of his or her emotions. Such a miserable wreck can also become cheerful, laughing, or manic, this transformation taking place overnight or even within a day. All these emotional ups and downs are quite devastating to patients, and also to their friends and families.

So there are two main causes of depression: one is the chemical imbalance in the brain interfering with normal brain cell function, the other is the reaction of anger and grief at developing M.E. In practice the causes cannot usually be isolated – what is important is to help the depressive symptoms.

There are other factors which may, if present, tip the scales between just coping and becoming depressed. These are:

- Exhaustion, which may precede a relapse
- Low blood sugar, which is treatable
- Candida overgrowth or sensitivity (there will probably be other symptoms to suggest this)
- Hormonal changes, for example premenstrual depression
- Food or chemical allergy reaction
- A personal upset
- Occasions like Christmas, which make many people depressed especially if they are lonely or ill
- Dark winter days

M.E. causes emotional fragility and a degree of paranoia.

When people or events make you upset, learn to say to yourself 'It doesn't matter, this can't hurt me.' Living with M.E. can *strengthen* our inner resources, and lead us to being less dependent on the opinions and approval of others. A friend with M.E. told me, 'I try not to react so much to upsetting things now, nor to get overexcited or overhappy. I have reduced the level of some of my emotional reactions and just let things wash past me, and it is easier to cope.'

It is easy for friends and family to cause hurt. You find out quickly who your real friends are; others melt away because they feel threatened by the illness. They do not know how to approach someone who has changed and whose mood may be unpredictable. The upset from such hurt can be lessened if you have a strong belief in yourself, and if you can realize that your *unique special self* (soul, spirit) *is still intact and special*, in spite of your being ill and losing friends.

Those with experience of depression can often recognize when they are going down-hill again. Before the thing has got hold of you and you don't have the will or insight to sort anything out, try looking to see if there is anything pulling you down which you can maybe change, or at least comprehend.

Early Signs of Depression Checklist

- Are you overdoing things? Extra rest and sleep, and letting go of striving, may help.
- Are you eating enough, and the right foods?
- If you are female, is your period due soon? If so, you know this bad bout will not last forever. Premenstrual depression is very common in women with M.E. (see page 247).
- If you have had symptoms pointing to candida overgrowth, could you be having a flare up, and need to take an antifungal agent and check your diet?
- Have you eaten something you normally avoid and to

which you may be hypersensitive, such as wheat? If so, this reaction will pass.

- Is there some extra chemical around, such as gas or new paint? If you cannot avoid it, take extra vitamin C and wait for the reaction to settle, or consider removing yourself from the new chemical, if possible.
- Is it a time of year when you have felt bad before? Many sufferers seem to find a seasonal pattern to their ups and downs. There is not much you can do about the earth turning, but at least you know it will go on turning and bring you to a better month. If it is winter, maybe a full-spectrum lamp will help if you cannot get outside.
- Weather can also influence mood. Damp weather seems to affect a lot of people; low pressure is associated with an increase in negative ions, and of moulds and fungal spores in the air.
- Is your low mood the result of some personal upset? If so, try and talk about it to someone you trust, instead of bottling it up.

It can happen that just when you think that the M.E. is receding, or that you have really got this illness sorted out and are coping wonderfully, then crash, down you go into a spell of depression and nothing you do seems to pull you out.

This happened to me last year, when I was trying to increase my exercise tolerance, and thought I was doing very well! I was very depressed for weeks, but came through it.

What now helps me most is (a) getting more physical and mental rest, (b) using either sleeping pills or low dose tricyclic antidepressants to ensure me a run of nights of sleep.

Each bout of depression I get *always* follows a period of extra activity, mental or physical, and comes with other symptoms of relapse – fever, sore throat, sweating, muscle twitching and pain, etc. This leads me to believe that most M.E. depression is a symptom of brain disturbance due to the disease.

So what encouragement can be offered to people going through a low patch? The following ideas may help carers as well as patients, and if you have M.E. and are at present well enough to read and understand this, then store this information up against a future bad time:

- Remember that *you*, a unique special person, are the same person underneath the depression. The essential you is intact, even when you feel disintegrated and cut off from the world. Try to see the depression as an awful symptom to be borne patiently until it passes.
- *This time of blackness will pass.* Be very patient with yourself, remember that seasons come and go, and so do moods.
- *Do not feel ashamed of being as you are.* Depression is a symptom of the illness, and may need treatment.
- Make a list (on paper or in your head) of all the people you have ever known who love you, and care about what happens to you. Do this while you are less depressed, and take this list out and refer to it if you have a bad time. Those people *still* care about you while you are depressed.

Allow those people who love you to give you their affection even if you cannot give anything back at the time. The thoughts and prayers of others can sustain you during a long bad patch. Michael Mayne, present Dean of Westminster and M.E. person, said 'When I was depressed I found I could not even pray, so I had to allow others to do the praying for me.'

Some of you may live alone, and may feel that you have no one who cares about you. There is probably someone, maybe at a distance, who could be contacted by phone or a written note. Could any friend fail to respond to a simple plea, such as 'I'm going through a very bad patch just now – please think of me, or phone me, or come and see me'? The British 'stiff upper lip' serves no purpose; admit you are low, and ask for help and reassurance.

The majority of those other people out there who appear to be happy and stable have probably gone through depression at some time in their lives. Those most able to understand and give support are those who have been in the dark valley and know what it is like. Such people may be contacted through your local support group, local church, or one of the national M.E. societies' telephone help-lines.

Try and give yourself treats, or allow others to pamper you. For instance, a nice warm bath with essential oils in, a new nightgown, something very good to eat, a visit from a hairdresser and some make-up, a new book or record, some beautiful flowers, or an outing if someone can take you. A problem of course is that if you have depression *and* M.E., you may be in physical relapse and not strong enough for outings. A trip to a garden where you can just sit and take in the gifts of nature might be more appropriate.

One of the classic features of depression is the loss of self-esteem. By trying to give yourself treats, you are reinforcing your affection for yourself. *There is nothing wrong with loving yourself.* Loving yourself is not the same as selfishness, it means accepting and caring about your individual personality with all its faults and weaknesses, just as you accept the imperfections of a loved friend.

Laughter is good medicine for any illness. In his book *Anatomy of an Illness*, Norman Cousins tells of how, when confronted by sudden, severe, life-shattering arthritis, he withdrew from life and watched comedies on videos for days. He laughed his way back to health.

One way to boost self-esteem is to manage to complete a small task each day. There is no point in setting impossible goals that you cannot achieve without collapse, so the task needs to be something within your grasp. Perhaps writing a short letter, tidying a drawer, or doing a small patch of weeding, according to your ability.

The positive feedback from accomplishing something, especially if you see the result, can give a small boost each day. A certain degree of apathy may need to be overcome, but it is amazing how once the initial effort is made, the concentration required overcomes the misery for a time. Do not set a goal which is beyond your powers; if the task is unreasonable you will give up half-way through, and this can be counterproductive.

Antidepressant Drugs?

Some M.E. sufferers have been helped by anti-depressants; others have been unable to tolerate them, or have found no benefit. Often when they are not tolerated, the drug has been prescribed in too high a dose.

The antidepressants called *tricyclics* (because of their chemical formula) were originally developed as antihistamines to treat allergies. The chemical formulae of the tricyclics and of the antihistamines used to treat hay fever and skin allergies are very similar. For this reason tricyclic antidepressants are sometimes used to treat chronic skin problems. Both of these formulae also closely resemble the formula of the phenothiazines used to treat schizophrenia and mania.

Tricyclics work by altering the available levels of some neuro-transmitters, with effects not only on mood, but on the transmission of other nerve impulses. So it is not surprising that brain functions in general may improve, such as memory, concentration, sleep patterns, and sensitivity to pain and noise. As these drugs also have antihistamine effects, they may modify some allergic symptoms as well.

Do not dismiss antidepressants if your doctor suggests this treatment, unless you have already tried them and were made worse.

Some may find their depression is helped by a nutritious diet, plus extra B vitamins, zinc and magnesium, and perhaps amino acids as a supplement. If antidepressants are prescribed, then those with the least side-effects should be used, and the smallest dose used to begin with.

The important thing to remember about anti-depressants is that they do not work overnight like aspirins or sleeping pills. It will be at least two weeks before you see any real improvement in your depression. But better sleep and lessened anxiety will come almost straight away, which can be a great relief if there is marked insomnia and agitation as well as depression.

The possible side-effects of tricyclics are: dry mouth, blurred vision, difficulty passing urine, constipation, low blood-pressure, dizziness, an irregular or slow heartbeat, and nightmares.

Most side-effects settle after the first week or two, especially if the dose is increased gradually.

The starting dose should be much smaller for an M.E. patient than would normally be prescribed.

For example: Prothiaden 25 mg at night, increasing to 50 or 75 mg. Trimiprimine 10 mg at night, increasing to 20 mg or more daily.

If you have unpleasant side-effects at the start of treatment, especially any heart symptoms or missed beats, tell your doctor. Some of the newer tricyclics have fewer side-effects.

Another antidepressant that is non-sedative, and therefore can be taken in the morning is called Prozac (Fluoxetine hydrochloride). It is used more in the USA than in the UK at present – many M.E. people in the UK have reported unpleasant side-effects.

The other main type of antidepressants, MAOIS, are not used as first choice. They interact with any foods that contain tyramine or other amines, and alarming rises in blood-pressure can occur. If you are put on MAOIS you will be given a list of all the dangerous foods, which include cheese and broad beans. This is one more hazard for an M.E. patient to contend with, and life is complicated enough without yet more foods to avoid.

From my own experience and that of many others, I find that the main benefit of tricyclic drugs in people with viral onset M.E. (rather than 'chronic fatigue') is that they help to improve sleep, and achieving this requires only a low dose. When the dose was increased, we felt worse and more depressed. What is urgently needed is a trial of tricyclic therapy for people with M.E., compared with the same treatment for people with depressive disorder but no M.E. features.

If you are getting better on antidepressants *do not suddenly stop them*. Even if you think you don't need them any more, you need to reduce the daily dose very gradually, under regular medical supervision. Sudden withdrawal could put you right back to where you started from, or even worse.

Sadly, there is a small but steady toll of people with M.E. who find they just cannot bear life any more, and take the only route left to them. Perhaps they would not have committed suicide if they had had someone who believed and supported them; if they had a sympathetic employer; if they had seen a doctor who had recognized the risk, placed them under supervision and started antidepressant treatment.

So please, if you, as a person with M.E., or if someone you know with M.E. is seriously depressed and has thought or talked of suicide, *do get medical help*, and don't refuse treatment or hospital admission if this is advised.

If you are not taking any nutritional supplements already, consider the following, all of which are necessary for good brain function:

Vitamin B complex, (or as part of a multivitamin), containing at least 20 mg each B_1, B_2, B_6; vitamin C, zinc, and magnesium; and amino acid complex, if you have poor food absorption.

Psychotherapy

The term psychotherapy is used here rather loosely, and refers to the sort of skilled help that can be given by a psychiatrist, a psychotherapist, a counsellor, or anyone else trained in this field.

Psychotherapy proper is not suggested for someone in the early acute stage of illness, nor during a relapse, because there just is not the energy available for the talking and self-understanding that is part of the therapy. Digging up past painful experiences does not help an ill person; better help comes from a skilled listener, and by dealing together with problems of the present moment.

Learning to live with a debilitating illness is difficult. One of the first steps to coping is accepting the illness and coming to terms with the limitations it imposes.

Anger and grief are perfectly normal reactions to developing a condition such as M.E. If these emotions can be expressed and admitted, instead of being suppressed and driven inside, then the patient has a better chance of maintaining a degree of sanity, and of coping with further relapses or depression.

Often, family and friends really want to help the M.E. sufferer, who they see is devastated by the symptoms and loss of normal life, but they may not have the skills needed to help psychologically. So seeing an outsider who has these skills (when you are not acutely ill or starting a relapse) is worth thinking about.

Loneliness

I have talked about grief and anger and their roles in contributing to depression. Loneliness is a feeling that hurts a lot of M.E. people, even those living in a family situation. Chronic illness may lose you friends, but it need not: a lot depends on how you view your friends and family. For example, if you become jealous of the health of others, this shows, and drives them away.

Self-pity, moaning about how unfair life is, and seeing yourself as a victim all lead in the end to resentment. *Much of life is unfair and difficult for every human being!* You and I have a strange illness, other people have different problems. Many people in the world are starving to death as you read this. Feelings of resentment, envy and self-pity can only make the illness worse, and they get between you and friends and lead to loneliness.

Past hurts and grievances, if they are hung onto, eat away inside and also cause resentment. All sorts of barriers that stop you loving other people, and keep their affection from you, can spring up from jealousy and resentment. Loneliness is partly a state of mind. People can feel lonely surrounded by a crowd in a city, or not feel lonely while apparently isolated in a deserted landscape.

The key to this is being content with yourself, liking yourself enough to want to have *you* as your friend.

I do not write these things as an outsider with no understanding – believe   me,   I   *still*   experience loneliness, envy of relatives who are fit and active, and anger. However, I think it is natural to feel these things. What is destructive is either not acknowledging these emotions, or feeding on them. Once you are aware of them, express them – on paper or out loud when alone! – then throw them away and replace them with more useful thoughts.

Here are some words by the writer Kahlil Gibran, taken from his little masterpiece *The Prophet*. They speak clearly about unhappiness and the pain of depression:

    . . . *Of Joy and Sorrow* . . .
    When you are joyous, look deep into your heart and you
    shall find it is only that which has given you sorrow that is
    giving you joy.
    When you are sorrowful, look again in your heart, and
    you shall see that in truth you are weeping for that which
    has been your delight.

Some of you say, 'Joy is greater than sorrow', and others say, 'Nay, sorrow is the greater.'

But I say unto you, they are inseparable.

Together they come, and when one sits alone with you at your board, remember that the other is asleep upon your bed.

. . . *Of Pain* . . .

Your pain is the breaking of the shell that encloses your understanding.

Even as the stone of the fruit must break, that its heart may stand in the sun, so must you know pain.

And could you keep your heart in wonder at the daily miracle of your life, your pain would not seem less wondrous than your joy;

And you would accept the seasons of your heart, even as you have always accepted the seasons that pass over your fields.

And you would watch with serenity through the winters of your grief.

Suggested Further Reading

Michael Mayne, *A Year Lost and Found*, (Darton, Longman and Todd, 1987).

M. Scott Peck, *The Road Less Travelled*, (Arrow Books, 1990).

Chapter 11

Good Nutrition for CFS and M.E.

Why is good nutrition so important for someone with M.E.?

- Because deficiencies of essential nutrients may have developed before the onset of M.E., due to poor diet or stress earlier in life.
- Because digestion and absorption of food may be impaired. This can result from damage to the lining of the small intestine, or a reduction of digestive enzymes due to an intestinal infection.
- Because the immune system needs a good supply of protein, essential fats, certain minerals and vitamins if it is to function efficiently.

Changing and improving diet is one of the simplest ways of effecting progress with M.E. A special anti-candida diet is described in Chapter 13.

Guidelines for Basic Healthy Eating

- Eat regular meals, do not miss breakfast or lunch.
- Use fresh, unprocessed foods as far as possible. Avoid dried, packaged, dehydrated, or canned food.
- Avoid refined carbohydrates – sugar (brown or white), white flour, polished rice, white pasta.
- Avoid alcohol, coffee, tea (except weak tea in moderation), cola drinks, chocolate.
- Have good-quality protein at least once a day.
- Have plenty of fresh fruit and vegetables.
- Have some raw vegetable in a salad every day. Vegetables – except potatoes and beans – should be

cooked lightly in a little water or steamed to conserve their vitamins and minerals.

- Peel or wash fruit with skins, and thoroughly wash all vegetables, unless you know they are organically grown. Try and use them as fresh as possible.
- Be more adventurous with salads, using sprouted legumes (e.g. bean sprouts), grated carrot, grated beetroot, shredded cabbage, etc. in winter when the more traditional salad foods are out of season. If you already possess a food-processor, you should make full use of it to prepare finely chopped salads and thick vegetable soups.
- If you can afford it, consider investing in a juicer, which extracts much more of the enzymes, vitamins and minerals from living plants than can be obtained by liquidizing or squeezing them. Highly nutritious drinks of fruit and vegetable juice can be made, leaving only the undigestible cellulose behind. You would need to eat a very large volume of these plants to get the equivalent amount of goodness you get from the juice. Juiced fruits or vegetables are ideal for someone with a poor appetite, or for someone who lives alone and is too ill to chop and peel food.

Vegetables and fruit are important, not only to supply a good daily level of vitamin C, but many other essential nutrients. If it can be digested, some raw food should be eaten daily, as vitamins and enzymes are partially destroyed by cooking. Irradiated foods, which may appear more fresh and attractive than non-irradiated fruits and vegetables (because they do not go mouldy and have a longer shelf life), are dead foods – their plant enzymes having been destroyed. Any value of consuming live, fresh plant food is lost by irradiation.

Protein

Protein is made up of amino acids. These are the building blocks used for repair and replacement of all body cells. They are also essential for making antibodies (which fight infection), neuro-transmitters, hormones, and the chemicals (lymphokines, or cytokines) produced by the immune system. Some amino acids can be made in our bodies; others must be supplied in food: these are called *essential amino acids*. For any diet to be adequate in its protein supply, it must supply enough of the essential amino acids.

So-called 'first-class' proteins contain all the essential amino acids in the right balance. These are proteins derived from animal sources: meats, fish, eggs, and dairy products.

Second-class proteins are deficient in one or more of the essential amino acids, and come from plants. However, by combining plant proteins properly, all the amino acids are supplied, e.g. rice with lentils, wheat with beans. This principle is used by vegans to construct an adequate diet.

Although meat is traditionally regarded as a good protein food, it does have drawbacks:

1. It can be high in animal fat, i.e. saturated fat, the kind we are not supposed to have too much of.
2. Unless you obtain meat from animals that have been organically reared, or from wild game, you risk consuming hormones and antibiotics which are added to animal feeds.

The best meats are:

- Organically-reared chicken and turkey.
- Venison, rabbit, pheasant and other game.
- Lamb – especially mountain lamb (sheep are usually free-ranging) – although this is not low in fat.
- Liver, heart, kidney etc. (offal) from organically-raised animals. These are low in fat and rich in other nutrients as well as in protein.

Meat is much more digestible if cooked long and slowly, as in a casserole.

Fish is an excellent food, it is a complete protein, easily digested, and contains fish oils, which supply essential fats. Fish is also a good source of iodine and zinc. Even if you don't normally eat it, try and have fish at least twice a week.

Eggs are another excellent food, because even though an average egg contains only 7–8 gm of protein, it is a complete protein and easily digested. They are also a good source of cholesterol, B vitamins, vitamins A and E, and zinc. Eggs from free-ranging chickens are additive-free, and better in flavour and nutrient content.

Milk and its products (if you are not milk-allergic) are also good sources of protein. Skimmed milk is better than full-cream milk as it has less fat and more protein and calcium per volume. The best cheeses are those which are low-fat and have no added yellow colour and no mould. Plain, live yoghourt is excellent as a source of protein and calcium, and has the bacteria needed for proper balance in the colon. Some people who are intolerant of cow's milk can tolerate yoghourt, goat's or sheep's milk.

In M.E., it is important to have a good intake of all essential amino acids for any recovery to take place. If the gut lining or pancreas have been affected by a virus, there may not be enough digestive enzymes to break down protein into small enough molecules to be absorbed. Because of this, some people find it helpful to take supplements of amino acids, especially if they have frequent digestive and bowel problems, plus severe psychological symptoms.

Is a vegetarian diet suitable for someone with M.E.? It depends on what you are used to, and how you feel on a high-meat diet. It is possible to have enough high-quality protein as a lactovegetarian (i.e. vegetables and dairy products). But a vegan diet relies exclusively on protein from grains, pulses, and nuts. This may be fine for those in perfect health, but many M.E. sufferers are intolerant of wheat, and also have problems digesting pulses in any quantity, due to a lack of digestive enzymes. So a diet of bread, rice and beans may cause extra bloating, pain, and gas. A vegan diet can also lead to deficiencies of essential amino acids, vitamins B_{12} and D, zinc, iron, and calcium. Soya products – soya milk, tofu – are used in a vegan diet and contain calcium and protein, however intolerance to soya develops easily in anyone with a tendency to allergies.

So, for all these reasons, a vegan diet is not recommended to anyone trying to get better from M.E.

It is not a good idea when you are ill to change suddenly from being a vegetarian to a flesh eater, or vice versa. Your digestive system and liver may not adapt very well, so any dietary changes should be made gradually.

Carbohydrates

These provide the main fuel for energy supply. Someone doing hard exercise daily, such as a labourer or athlete, needs plenty of carbohydrates to burn. An M.E. sufferer will need much less.

Refined carbohydrates are pure starch or sugar, from which the husk and germ have been largely removed by refining. They are quickly digested and absorbed, but tend to lead to a to rapid rise in blood glucose level; this is followed in two to three hours by a drop in blood glucose, which may give the unpleasant symptoms of low blood-sugar (see below).

Refined carbohydrates provide 'empty calories' – calories but no other nutrients, and little fibre. Valuable B vitamins, minerals, vegetable oils and fibre are removed in the milling process.

Complex carbohydrates are the starch together with the husk and seed-germ, such as wholewheat, unrefined oats, brown rice, other wholegrains, and potatoes with their skins. They are more slowly digested, leading to a gradual rise in blood glucose. With complex carbohydrates you have to eat a lot more in volume to give the same amount of energy as refined carbohydrate. To get 250 calories of energy, is it healthier to eat a small bar of chocolate, or four slices of wholemeal bread?

Sugar is called 'pure, white, and deadly', with good reason. It is a relatively recent addition to the diet of humans. The high consumption of sugar in sweets, cakes, breakfast cereals and canned drinks is responsible not only for tooth decay, but for obesity, diabetes, heart disease, and many other disorders. Honey is still a sugar, but marginally better, as it contains minute amounts of minerals and vitamins.

Hypoglycaemia

Low blood-sugar (hypoglycaemia) can be overlooked as a cause of many symptoms, which result not only from the blood-sugar being low, but also from blood-sugar levels falling too rapidly. Blood-sugar control may be faulty in M.E. sufferers due to involvement of the hypothalamus, where many controls of the body are situated.

After a meal is eaten there is a steady rise in blood-sugar level as the food is digested and absorbed into the bloodstream. This triggers off release of the sugar-controlling hormone *insulin*, produced by certain cells in the pancreas. The insulin lowers blood-sugar by pushing glucose into cells, but if a load of glucose is absorbed from the gut quickly, as happens if a meal high in sugar is eaten (e.g. two bars of chocolate), a lot of insulin is released and there may be an overreactive fall in blood-sugar level, giving symptoms.

Symptoms Produced by a Rapid Fall in Blood Glucose

- Feeling faint or dizzy, nausea, sweating, pallor
- Rapid, weak pulse
- Feeling 'spaced out', irritability

- Irrational, bizarre behaviour (like someone drunk)
- Headache, poor concentration, panic attacks, inability to make decisions
- Slurred speech, blurred vision
- Fatigue, muscle weakness, unsteady gait
- Insomnia, waking in the night hungry and not being able to go back to sleep without eating

Any of these symptoms may occur. The earliest signs are hunger, faintness and an inability to think straight. The most common times these signs arise are 11 a.m.–1 p.m. and 4–6 p.m., from two to four hours following a meal. If hunger itself is not present, then it may be easy to overlook hypoglycaemia as a cause of feeling unwell. If eating a meal or having a sweet drink banishes symptoms, this suggests that low blood-sugar was present.

Many people who feel terrible first thing in the morning reach for a cup of coffee not just as a stimulant, but because caffeine boosts blood-sugar – for a short time only; by 10 a.m. they are usually irritable and desperate for the next cup of coffee. Probably most accidents occur at work mid- to late morning and late afternoon, and many road accidents may be caused by low blood-sugar. How often do family rows flare up just before mealtimes?

We who live in wealthy countries have more than we need to eat, so how is it that hunger and low blood-sugar cause so many people to feel unwell so much of the time? For this problem is extremely common, as any of you who have irritable spouses and whining children at the end of the afternoon will know.

Most attacks of hypoglycaemia are rebound drops which follow a too-rapid rise in blood-sugar.

Common Causes of Reactive Hypoglycaemia

1. Consumption of refined carbohydrates, i.e. sugar, honey, sweets, chocolate, cakes, soft drinks, etc.

There is a trend towards eating snacks instead of balanced meals; the snacks are often high in sugar, salt or fat, with little real nutritional value. These non-foods can produce a rapid rise in blood glucose, giving a temporary lift for an hour, followed by hypo-glycaemic symptoms. So the binger on sweet things has violent swings in blood-sugar through the day, with parallel mood changes. The long-term result of this can sometimes be pancreatic exhaustion and diabetes.

2. A reaction to an allergenic food, e.g. wheat.

   Hypoglycaemia may be a symptom of food allergies, and if the symptoms do not improve after following dietary advice, then food allergy should be suspected.

3. Consumption of coffee, tea, alcohol – caffeine and alcohol both stimulate the release of sugar stored in the liver without replacing it. Much of an alcoholic hangover is due to low blood-sugar, the best cure for which is a hearty breakfast rather than coffee and aspirin. People who need coffee or tea many times a day are reactive hypoglycaemics as well as caffeine addicts.

4. Nicotine also stimulates a rise in blood-sugar from liver reserves. Tobacco is no good for M.E. anyway.

5. Candida yeast overgrowth seems to lead to haywire sugar control. One theory proposed is that the yeast gobbles up the digested carbohydrate sugars, preventing their absorption, but this is hard to prove. Those who improve on an anti-candida regime usually find their blood-sugar control improves.

6. Stress, if prolonged, can cause low blood-sugar (see Chapter 9).

7. Hormonal disturbance. Many women find their sugar control worse in the 10 days or so premenstrually; this contributes to premenstrual tension and depression.

8. Nutritional deficiencies. Deficiencies of vitamin B_6, chromium, zinc, manganese, magnesium, and other B vitamins can all increase the likelihood of hypo-

glycaemia. These nutrients are involved in the hormonal and chemical glucose-control mechanisms.

Ways of Avoiding Hypoglycaemia

1. Eat regular meals, if necessary eat four, five or six smaller meals instead of two or three per day. Try and stick to a regular pattern; the body clock comes to expect food at particular times, and delaying a meal by an hour or more can bring on symptoms.

2. Eat a decent breakfast, probably the most important meal of the day for a low blood-sugar person. A cup of coffee and a slice of toast is not much to combat overnight starvation, yet millions of workers expect to get a morning's work done on just that. If you can't face food first thing, have some fruit and something more substantial a bit later.

3. Avoid sugar and refined starches. The answer to low blood-sugar is not to have a lot of sugar, which perpetuates the problem, but rather food that provides a more gradual rise in blood-sugar. Have more protein, with low-carbohydrate meals, or else have more complex carbohydrates. Sugar-free muesli for breakfast will provide more protein, and fibre, than cornflakes or white bread; it takes longer to be digested and gives a more gradual blood-sugar rise.

However, for M.E. sufferers, there is an exception to this no sugar rule: you may need a boost to your blood-sugar if you suddenly become faint, sweaty and near collapse between meals. On such an occasion, eating two biscuits or sucking some glucose sweets will revive you enough so you can get home, or get to the kitchen to obtain something more substantial. This emergency measure may be essential if you get an attack of hypoglycaemic symptoms, especially if away from the house. This is not the same behaviour as regularly eating bars of chocolate or having sweet puddings. In spite of my anti-sugar propaganda, I try to remember to keep some glucose sweets or fruit in my handbag for emergencies.

Fats

Fats delay absorption of food. The classic British breakfast of eggs and bacon lasts all morning, as compared with cornflakes or toast. Bacon may not be ideal, but having eggs, or extra butter or margarine, or a little pure vegetable oil added to muesli, may be helpful.

Night Hunger

If you are a kitchen-raider at 3 a.m., have your evening meal later, or have a pre-bedtime mini-meal – a milky drink late in the evening can be helpful, so long as milk is not a problem. Keep biscuits or crispbread or a sandwich ready on your bedside table.

Avoid caffeine, cola, alcohol, and nicotine.

Remember that continuing mental or emotional stress lowers blood-sugar.

Nutritional Supplements to Help Blood-sugar Control

The regime suggested on page 168 should provide all necessary nutrients. It may be worth taking a chromium supplement such as chromium GTF (200 micrograms daily), although a good multivitamin and mineral pill should contain some chromium. Chromium GTF, plus all the B vitamins, have been found to benefit both hypoglycaemia and diabetes. The best natural source of chromium is brewer's yeast, which is fine so long as you are not yeast allergic (see page 178 in Chapter 13).

Not all people with M.E. have hypoglycaemia, and not all hypoglycaemics have M.E. There is quite a lot of overlap in the symptoms, though, and the likelihood of having an unstable blood-sugar seems to be high among M.E. patients, especially during a relapse. M.E. people most at risk of low blood-sugar attacks are those who *continue to do too much*, those who cannot reduce stress levels, and those who eat badly or infrequently.

Fats

We are being urged to reduce our fat consumption as part of a healthier diet. What is more important is to change the *balance*, to have more essential fats and less saturated fats, which are mostly of animal source.

Essential Fatty Acids (EFAs)

These are found in good-quality, polyunsaturated vegetable oils and margarines, nuts and seeds, most vegetables, and in fish, especially oily fish.

They are essential for life and cannot be manufactured in the body, so have to be eaten in the diet. Apart from needing fat as a store of available energy and for insulation, we need essential fatty acids because they form the main structure of cell membranes and walls in every body cell; they are also needed to make highly active substances which are vital for all body functions. 80 per cent of the white matter of the brain is made from essential fatty acids; nerves have an insulating coat, called the *myelin sheath*, also composed of the same fatty acids. (Hence the old saying 'fish is good for your brain').

Fatty acids are divided broadly into two groups, called *saturated* and *unsaturated*. The saturated fats tend to be hard, are found in meat, lard, cheese, butter, hardened margarines, and overheated oils.

The unsaturated fats tend to be liquid or soft at normal temperatures. When unsaturated fats (e.g. vegetable oil) are heated they take on hydrogen atoms and become saturated, hence losing their value.

It is the *imbalance* of too much saturated fat in relation to unsaturated that leads to deposition of excess fats inside blood-vessel walls, which leads to heart disease, high blood-pressure, strokes, etc. Eskimos living on their natural diet, which is very high in fish oil, are renowned for their low rate of obesity and lack of the diseases known to most Western societies, in spite of a high level of total fats in their diet. They are protected because of the unsaturated fats in fish oils.

Processed vegetable oils and hardened margarines are actually worse for you than butter or cream, because they contain types of saturated fatty acids that block the body's utilization of the good, essential fats. Not all polyunsaturated fats are essential fatty acids. The important EFAs are linoleic acid, linolenic acid, and those derived from fish oils.

So why all this emphasis on EFAs in M.E.?

Essential fatty acids are needed to make, among other things, *prostaglandins*, which have very important functions.

There are numerous types of prostaglandins, and their function is to regulate the biochemistry and enzyme activities of all body cells. They are very active, but very short-lived. There are many prostaglandins, one in particular is of interest in M.E.: it is called *PGE1*, and is derived from linoleic acid, an essential fat present in vegetable oils.

Some of PGE1 Functions (relevant to M.E.)

Improves circulation of blood
Lowers blood-pressure
Restores normal shape and movement of red blood cells
Inhibits inflammation
Activates T lymphocytes in immune system
Has effects on transmission at nerve endings and nerve
  conduction

PGE1 is found to be low in diabetics, people suffering hardening of the arteries or many psychiatric disorders, and in allergic people.

There are various things which may block the synthesis of PGE1 from linoleic acid, and cause a lack of this important prostaglandin. These include:

Deficiency of zinc, magnesium, biotin, vitamin B_6 alcohol, chemicals, diabetes, and *viral infections*

The block in the stages from linoleic acid to PGE1 can be bypassed if gamma linolenic acid – known as *GLA*, and one of the substances made en route – is supplied directly in the diet. GLA occurs naturally in certain seeds, especially the seeds of the evening primrose and blackcurrants, the main sources of commercially-prepared GLA supplements.

So, from knowing that viral infections can block production of PGE1, one can understand why, in chronic and persistent viral infections, many symptoms develop due to lack of PGE1, especially allergies.

Linoleic acid makes another prostaglandin, called PGE2, via arachidonic acid, which also occurs in meat.

The PGE2 series have different actions to PGE1, that is, harmful ones: They make smooth muscle contract and promote platelet stickiness – platelets are the tiny cells in the blood that form clots. They also produce inflammation, reddening of skin, and swelling – all unpleasant symptoms.

Arachidonic acid, a product of linoleic acid, itself leads to inflammation.

So, if a diet is high in arachidonic acid (meat) but low in linoleic acid (vegetables), there will tend to be greater production of the pro-inflammatory PGE2 series and less of the anti-inflammatory PGE1 series. A diet with a greater amount of vegetables and fish relative to meat will tend to produce relatively more of the PGE1 prostaglandins, hence less inflammation, allergies or clotting.

Prostaglandin 3 series and related substances are formed from alpha-linolenic acid, found in beans, wheat and spinach, and from eicosapentaenoeic acid (EPA), found mainly in fish oils. The PG3 series are important in preventing thrombosis.

It is currently thought that a combination of essential

fatty acids from vegetable oils, nuts and seeds, and those in fish oils, is best for health.

This can be achieved by eating generous amounts of a wide range of vegetables, including green leafy vegetables daily, having about four teaspoons daily of a pure unrefined vegetable oil (cold-pressed olive oil is best), for example as a dressing on salads, using a high-quality unsaturated margarine, avoiding oil used for deep frying (better to use a little olive oil for occasional frying), and eating fish two or three times a week. The best fish are herring, mackerel, sardine, tuna, whitebait, shellfish, and roe.

Some people may need to take supplements of EFAs, primarily of gamma linoleic acid (GLA), which is marketed as oil of evening primrose or blackcurrant seed oil. This is recommended for M.E. sufferers, especially if they have become allergic.

Recent research (Behan, 1990) has shown that people with M.E. benefit from taking EFA supplements. The supplement needs to contain GLA and fish oil – e.g. *Efamol Marine* – and a minimum of 3 grams per day is recommended.

Fluids

In an average day, someone may drink four cups of coffee, three cups of tea, a glass or two of wine or a pint of beer, and perhaps a can of sweet fizzy drink. All these contain too much caffeine, as well as possibly sugar.

What is wrong with water? Many people rarely drink it, and the chemical chlorinated taste of most tap water is certainly off-putting. Water tastes better if it is spring water, or is filtered. Chlorine, lead, copper, nitrates and most agrochemicals can be removed from tap water by using a domestic water filter. An average person should drink at least two pints (a litre) of water a day in one form or another, in addition to the fluid already in food, and much more in hot weather or if ill.

During a M.E. relapse or period of severe illness it is advisable to increase daily fluid intake to four pints (two litres) or more by drinking warm water between meals. This will help the kidneys to flush out toxins and other products of the body's reaction to the virus.

Many M.E. people have digestive problems due to a lack of digestive enzymes and stomach acid. If you drink fluids with, or just after, your meal, the digestive juices are diluted and digestion is weakened. It is better to drink fluids *between* main meals, i.e. at least half an hour before or two hours after.

Fibre

Fibre is the indigestible residue (celluloses, pectins, gums and mucilages) composed of cell walls in plant foods, which passes right through the intestines and forms part of the faeces. It has no nutritional value of itself, but it is essential to provide bulk in the large intestine (colon). Its chief property is absorbing water, making a bulky stool which passes more quickly and smoothly through the colon to the rectum for evacuation.

Lack of fibre may result in:

- Constipation. Besides being uncomfortable, constipation contributes to piles, varicose veins, and undesirable effects of food residues remaining too long in the colon – fermentation, absorption of toxins, etc.
- Diverticulitis, gallstones
- A higher risk of cancer of the colon
- Too high a level of cholesterol (hence risk of heart disease)
- Alteration in the balance of the bacteriae in the colon, which may favour overgrowth of undesirable bugs, such as candida albicans. This imbalance is called *dysbiosis*, and may be implicated in many other illnesses.

In spite of much publicity, wheat bran is not the best source of fibre. It may cause problems – bloating, gas, pain, a spastic colon – in people who are wheat intolerant, which includes many M.E. sufferers. Wheat fibre is also high in *phytates*, which inhibit absorption of magnesium, calcium, iron and zinc. Phytates are only a problem in added wheat bran or in unleavened bread, and are broken down in the leavening process of normal bread.

The best sources of fibre are a high intake of mixed fruits and vegetables, wholegrains (including oats and unrefined rice), and some pulses.

Advice is given in later chapters about special anti-candida and allergy diets. To summarize, here are the guidelines for a basic healthy diet:

Include	*Avoid If Possible*
Complex carbohydrates (wholegrains, brown rice)	Additives, colourings
	Sugar, refined starches
	Alcohol, cola, caffeine
Fish	Processed meats
Lean meat, poultry, game, organ meats (liver, etc.)	Foods high in animal fat
	Tinned fruit
Eggs (free range), milk, low-fat cheese, yoghourt	Pastry, fried foods
Lots of fresh vegetables	
Mixed salad once or twice daily	
Nuts and seeds (e.g. in muesli)	
Potatoes	
Fresh fruit	
Pulses in moderation (if tolerated)	
Pure vegetable oils	

Use fresh ingredients where possible, and organically-reared meat if obtainable. Wash all vegetables well. Eat regular meals, maybe four or five small meals a day if there is any tendency to low blood-sugar.

Do not spend valuable energy travelling long distances to buy organic food, unless you have a freezer to make a bulk buy of meat worthwhile. In an ideal situation, it would be best for all M.E. people (and indeed the whole population) to eat food that is 100 per cent free from chemicals. There is a greater awareness now about the hazards of chemicals, and many supermarkets label foods that are organically produced; it is also worth asking your local retailers if they can obtain organically-grown food.

However, some organic vegetable produce is very expensive, and if imported may not be fresh, and mouldy food is even worse than non-organic fresh food.

Suggested Further Reading

Adelle Davis, *Let's Get Well*, (Thorsons, 1992).

Stephen Davies and Alan Stewart, *Nutritional Medicine*, (Pan Books, 1987).

Leslie and Susannah Kenton, *Raw Energy*, (Century Arrow, 1986).

——, *Raw Energy Recipes*, (Arrow Books, 1989).

Chapter 12

Nutritional Supplements

This is a controversial subject. Some argue that if you eat a well-balanced diet of good, fresh foods, then it should not be necessary to take extra vitamins or minerals. For someone in perfect health this is probably true.

However, the Recommended Daily Allowance (RDA) for each nutrient is calculated for the average adult of average weight, in health, and is often the amount which is just sufficient to prevent deficiency disease. The RDA may be much less than the amount required for optimum health, and in disease states the body's requirements may increase dramatically to a level which cannot be met by a normal diet, particularly if there is reduced appetite or digestion.

Many M.E. patients have problems with digestion and absorption of food. Signs suggesting this are:

- Weight loss in spite of good food intake
- Stools that contain undigested food
- Stools that float, and difficult to flush away
- Diarrhoea, distension, abdominal pains

If you have these symptoms, especially weight loss with a good appetite, assume that you are not getting the full value from what you eat. As well as losing protein and fats, you may be losing calcium, iron, zinc, folic acid, vitamin B_{12}, and the fat-soluble vitamins A, E and D. Poor appetite or nausea will also lead to nutritional insufficiency. Even when there is fluctuating weight gain, nutrition may be poor, as sudden weight gain in M.E. is usually due to fluid retention.

Possible Causes of Poor Absorption in M.E.

- Virus infections may cause flattening of the microvilli (tiny projections) on the surface of cells lining the small intestine, hence loss of absorptive surface.
- If the pancreas has been involved in a present or earlier virus infection, there may be reduced production of pancreatic digestive enzymes.
- There may be overactivity of the gut in general, leading to the food being rushed through the small bowel, with too little time there for digestion and absorption. This overactivity results from an upset control of the autonomic nervous system, part of a hypothalamic disorder.

Aside from the digestion/absorption factors, M.E./CFS is now known to be a disease that causes excessive cytokine production, which is known to produce blocks in vitamin utilization, so extra vitamins are needed to overcome this defect in their use in the body.

Supplements may also be needed to provide enough of the nutrients that are essential for the body's immune system, nervous system and the various glandular functions.

In addition, even before the onset of M.E. there may have been some nutritional deficiencies, due to earlier poor diet, or maybe prenatally from poor maternal health.

So, for all these reasons, it is logical to take whatever is necessary to restore the body to health. It may also be safer to correct nutritional imbalances than to take drugs, which only modify the symptoms instead of treating the underlying cause of illness.

A problem for many M.E. people who are trying to decide about supplements is cost. A few (e.g. evening primrose oil) can be obtained on prescription, if your doctor can be persuaded that this is worthwhile. Otherwise, it helps to work out how much the supplements are going to cost per day, then to see what can be given up to pay for this. There are less important things in life, for example, the cost of newspapers . . . Like a lot of decisions with M.E., it is a matter of deciding on priorities.

Digestive Enzymes

If you or your doctor think you have poor absorption of food due to lack of digestive enzymes, then taking a preparation of these makes sense. They are obtainable on prescription, and are all made from pancreatic extract, with various trade names, e.g. *Pancrex*, *Nutrizyme*. The preparation may be in granules or powder, and should be taken just before or with a meal, as it is inactivated by stomach acid.

Hydrochloric Acid

The stomach normally secretes digestive juices containing hydrochloric acid in response to and in anticipation of food. In allergic people or those with chronic viral illness, fevers, diabetes, or rheumatoid arthritis, there is frequently *achlorhydria* – lack of gastric acid. This may lead to fermentation in the stomach, bad breath, gas, and poor digestion, especially of protein. The enzyme *pepsin* needs acid to work properly to start digesting protein. Acidity is also needed to absorb calcium and iron.

Hydrochloric acid can be taken in various preparations, on prescription, starting with a small dose with meals. (But *not* by those with proven overacidity or symptoms of an ulcer, so consult your doctor first.)

Vitamin C

This is one of the most essential vitamins to help you with M.E. It is not stored in the body, and is needed daily in food. A cytokine, interleukin 2, when infused into cancer patients produced a vitamin C-deficiency state by suppression of vitamin-C utilization. For this reason alone M.E. patients should take extra vitamin C.

What Does Vitamin C Do?

Vitamin C (ascorbic acid) is needed to make *collagen*, the fibrous framework of most of the body. It is vital for the continuous repair and regeneration of body tissues. It is also used by the adrenal gland to make the hormones noradrenaline, and cortisol. The adrenal gland in health is rich in ascorbic acid.

Vitamin C is a powerful anti-oxidant – it mops up free radicals of oxygen which are released in various biochemical reactions, and which may cause cell damage.

Vitamin C has important effects on the immune system: it promotes the formation of lymphocytes, lymphocyte mobility, and phagocytosis – some white cells can engulf and destroy bacteria and dead cells. They can only be efficient at this if they contain ascorbic acid. It is also involved in the manufacture of antibodies (immunoglobulins).

In addition, vitamin C acts as an antiviral agent, and in high doses activates T lymphocytes. In 1979, at the National Cancer Institute, USA (Pauling, 1986), an investigation found that giving vitamin C (5 gm per day) to healthy people aged 18–30 led to doubling the rate of formation of new lymphocytes.

An increased intake of vitamin C also leads to greater production of interferon. Interferons are proteins with anti-viral activity, produced by virus-infected cells.

Vitamin C inhibits the synthesis of PGE2 prostaglandins, and therefore reduces the pain and swelling these chemicals cause.

Much valuable work on the use of high-dose vitamin C to treat infections, cancer, and many disorders of immunity such as rheumatoid arthritis has been done by Dr Linus Pauling. While many sceptics have dismissed his work, Pauling argues that in tests where people took vitamin C and no benefit was found, they did not take a large enough dose. The RDA of vitamin C in Britain is 30 mg (obtained from half an orange!), but a more realistic minimum amount for good health would be 100 mg, and much more in illness.

Much of Dr Pauling's reasoning for a greater need of vitamin C comes from his calculations of the amounts of various nutrients in the diet of our ancestors. As man evolved he became unable to make vitamin C in the body, as most other mammals do, so he would only have survived by having enough in daily food. The daily amount of food that a hunter-gatherer would have needed to keep him active would have contained about 3 gm of vitamin C – a hundred times the modern 'daily allowance'. Early man's diet had a much greater ratio of raw fruits, vegetables, nuts and berries than that of a twentieth-century Western diet; however his total calorie intake was very poor by our standards.

Someone with an infection, undergoing major surgery, or in emotional shock needs far more vitamin C than 100 mg a day. It is used up by the adrenal glands in response to stress; wound-healing requires extra vitamin C, and it is used by the immune system to fight infection.

Vitamin C cannot be stored in the body, and any that is not used is excreted in the urine. The main undesirable effect from taking more than is needed is diarrhoea. This is why the term 'bowel tolerance' is used when advising people how much to take.

It is suggested that you take vitamin C in divided doses rather than one large dose, and start with 1 gm daily (500 mg in the morning and 500 mg in the evening). Increase this by 1 gm daily until you have loose bowel motions, then cut it back to 1 gm less. Because of the occasional risk of increased formation of kidney stones, the total daily dose should never exceed 9 gm, and should always be taken in divided doses and with plenty of fluids. Most

M.E. people do not need more than 3 gm daily except at times of unavoidable extra stress – e.g. when they have a bacterial infection or are about to undergo surgery. People with a history of kidney stones should take no more than 1 gm daily.

Pure vitamin C is ascorbic acid, a weak acid, but still an acid. The cheapest way to get it is as pure ascorbic acid powder from a supplier. One level teaspoon of powder is about 3 gm. It should be completely dissolved in water or fruit juice, and taken with or just after food to avoid irritating the stomach (which it rarely does). To counter the acidity, a little bicarbonate of soda can be added. (For supplier see Appendix A.)

Vitamin C can be also taken as calcium ascorbate, or in buffered 1 gm tablets which dissolve in water to make a fizzy drink. The latter are more expensive.

Vitamin B_6 – Pyridoxine

Vitamin B_6 is important in many chemical processes, including the production and reactions of brain chemicals, which affect mood and behaviour, and in the pathways of essential fatty acids (EFAs), which are needed for the immune system. B_6 is needed for some minerals to work, especially magnesium.

Signs of lack of vitamin B_6 are: Depression, irritability, and red, greasy, scaly skin on the face. However, a lack of vitamin B_6 alone is unusual – there is usually a multiple B vitamin deficiency.

The recommended supplement level is about 20 mg daily, as part of a B-complex preparation. Women with premenstrual syndrome (PMS, see page 247) benefit from 50 mg daily during the premenstrual week.

All the B vitamins work and interact together, so individual B supplements are not recommended, apart from the extra B_6 before a period.

Vitamin B_{12}

This is normally only required in small amounts daily, about 1 microgm (mcg). It is found in meat, fish, and eggs; vegans risk a deficiency of it. As it is absorbed in the small intestine and needs a substance secreted by the stomach to combine with before absorption, people with deficient stomach juice or malabsorption in the small intestine are at risk of B_{12} deficiency. It is concerned with red cell production, and with nervous system functions. B_{12} deficiency can lead to anaemia, abnormal fatigue, pins and needles in the feet, stumbling gait, and mental confusion.

It is worthwhile for chronic M.E. sufferers to have their blood B_{12} level checked, especially if these neurological symptoms are prominent, if there are digestive/absorption problems, and if the patient is middle-aged or elderly. With the current publicity about M.E., there may well be people who think they have M.E., especially in the older age group, who in fact have a vitamin B_{12} deficiency, which is easily treatable.

Some M.E. sufferers do report an improvement in energy level and in neurological symptoms from B_{12} injections, although no clinical trials have yet been done. Dr Paul Cheney, of Charlotte NC, USA, uses vitamin B_{12} as part of his treatment regime, especially for treating fatigue. He recommends a trial dose of 3 mg twice a week (by injection). If there is a response, patients usually report improvement after two weeks, then can continue self-injecting 2–3 mg weekly. Dr Cheney says, 'We do not understand exactly why B_{12} works in CFS . . . an effect lasting only a few days does not fit in with normal B_{12} pharmokinetics. High-dose B_{12} must trigger some other effect, that lasts longer than the B_{12} itself' (Cheney, 1991).

The best sources of B_{12} (providing it is being absorbed) from food are liver, other organ meats and brewer's yeast (if tolerated; many cannot take yeast – see Chapter 13).

A good vitamin B-complex should be yeast-free and contain all the B vitamins, as follows:

Thiamine B_1
Riboflavin B_2
Pyridoxine B_6
    (about 10–20 mg daily for each of these)
Niacin B_3
Pantothenate B_5
Cyanocobalamin B_{12}
Folic acid
Para Amino Benzoic Acid (PABA)
Biotin

Information about the functions of other B vitamins, which are all needed, as they are interdependent, can be found in books about nutrition.

Vitamin A

Vitamin A itself occurs in animal produce; the best sources are animal and fish livers, kidneys, eggs and milk products. Beta-carotene, a precursor of vitamin A, is obtained from vegetables, particularly carrots, and other green-, yellow- or orange-coloured plants.

It is needed for maintaining mucous membranes, skin, and cell membranes, and is important in resisting infections. Vitamin A is one of the 'anti-oxidants' (along with vitamins C and E, and selenium), and therefore prevents damage to cell membranes, and has an important role in cancer prevention.

Vitamin A deficiency is one of the most common causes of blindness in poor countries, especially in small children, as a result of a poor diet.

As it is fat-soluble, and stored in the body, very high doses can accumulate and cause toxicity. Doses of up to 20,000 units daily are safe, but 7–15,000 units a day are sufficient unless there are particular indications of deficiency. The best way to supplement vitamin A is as part of a balanced multi-vitamin preparation, or in fish- or liver-oil capsules, which also provide essential fatty acids.

Pantothenic Acid (Vitamin B₅)

This little known vitamin is one of the B family. It occurs widely in many foods; it is essential for the proper function of adrenal glands, and for making antibodies. It is one of the anti-stress vitamins and is important for fighting infection and allergies.

It is present in most B-complex preparations. It seems to be helpful in high doses in stress-related diseases and in conditions where the immune system is not working properly, such as allergies or rheumatoid arthritis. It is recommended for M.E., and can be taken as calcium pantothenate in doses of 300–1,000 mg.

The symptoms of pantothenic acid deficiency (produced in volunteers) are remarkably similar to those of M.E. and of multiple allergies. It has even been suggested that members of families who are all allergic may have some inherited increased need for this vitamin.

Vitamin E

This is another fat-soluble vitamin, and most important for its anti-oxidant properties (like A, C, and selenium). It occurs in vegetables, nuts and eggs, and the recommended supplement is 100–200 IU daily. It is essential for proper wound-healing.

What Do Anti-oxidants Do?

Oxygen is essential for cells to live. However, in certain circumstances oxygen produces toxic derivatives, which can combine with other molecules and cause damage to cells and alter their function, or cause them to become cancerous, or to die. These nasty oxygen products are called 'free radicals', and are mopped up and made safe by anti-oxidants. Anti-oxidants are vitamins A, C, and E, and various enzymes that contain trace elements such as selenium, zinc, manganese, and copper. The free radicals cause damage to the fatty acid part of cell walls.

Free radicals have multiple sources, including chemicals in air pollution and food, and cigarette smoke, but are also produced by lymphocytes in inflammation, e.g. when the lymphocytes are killing virus-infected cells.

In M.E., there seems to be a persistent low-grade viral infection, and disordered cell functions all over the body. Some doctors have used the term 'sick cell syndrome' about M.E. So it seems logical to minimize damage to the cells from free radicals by ensuring a good intake of the nutrients needed for a good anti-oxidant system.

Zinc

Zinc is a trace element which is necessary for a wide range of chemical reactions in the body. Studies of zinc and its many roles have begun relatively recently, and there is still much to discover.

Signs of a Zinc Deficiency

- impaired wound-healing
- loss of sense of taste or smell
- slow growth
- infertility
- hair loss
- skin problems (including acne)
- allergies
- poor resistance to infection
- depression and other mental disturbances
- white spots on nails

Those at Risk of Zinc Deficiency

- Those with a poor intake of zinc due to:

a vegan diet
slimming
a strict allergy diet
poor appetite
being elderly
suffering from alcoholism
undergoing intravenous feeding
• Those who suffer poor absorption due to:
a high-fibre diet with lots of bran
low stomach acid
lack of pancreatic enzymes
iron tablets
• Malabsorption: due to gluten sensitivity (coeliac disease)

The daily requirement is about 15 mg for a healthy adult; more in pregnancy; much more after major surgery, burns, or any severe stress.

The assessment of zinc status is not satisfactory at present. Levels measured in blood plasma, urine or hair do not seem to be accurate. The blood level can vary enormously throughout a 24-hour period. The most reliable method of measurement is by analysis of sweat, but this requires specialist apparatus. A rough estimate of body zinc status can be done by a patient, using the fact that taste becomes dulled in zinc deficiency. A solution of zinc is swilled round the mouth, and if a sharp bitter taste develops afterwards, the zinc status is probably near normal. If there is little or no taste, zinc is low or very low. This test is commercially available; it is called *Test-Zinc*.

Since in M.E. there is immune dysfunction and probably persistent virus infection, also maybe poor digestion and absorption of food, it is sensible to take extra zinc. A zinc supplement is best not taken with food, since its absorption is inhibited by various foods. A preparation giving 20–50 mg elemental zinc, as zinc ororate, zinc sulphate, or amino chelated zinc, can be taken at bedtime.

Therapists with access to accurate assessment of zinc levels (e.g. Biolab of London) report that almost every M.E. patient tested is low in zinc.

Magnesium

Magnesium is absolutely vital for normal cell function. It is present inside every living cell as well as in teeth and bones. The correct balance of calcium and magnesium across cell membranes is essential for transmission of nerve impulses, and for muscle contraction and relaxation. Magnesium is also involved in many enzyme systems and chemical reactions in the body.

Magnesium occurs naturally in hard water, in whole grains, green vegetables, nuts and beans. A deficiency is most likely in someone on a poor diet, living in a soft water area, or with poor intestinal absorption.

Magnesium Deficiency Leads to

- Many neurological symptoms, tingling and numbness
- Poor co-ordination of limbs
- Muscle weakness, muscle cramps or twitching
- Heart rhythm abnormalities
- Hyperactivity in children
- Mental confusion
- Depression
- Anorexia, nausea, constipation

Many features of M.E. are similar to magnesium deficiency. In a recently published trial, Dr David Dowson and colleagues at Southampton University (Cox et al., 1991), found that magnesium in red blood cells of M.E. (designated CFS) patients is low. 20 patients and 20 matched controls were used. Average red cell magnesium for patients was significantly lower than for the controls. In a double-blind treatment trial, magnesium sulphate was given by intramuscular injection weekly for 6 weeks to 17 of 34 M.E. subjects. The others received 2 ml water injections. At the end of the trial 80 per cent of those who had magnesium had significant improvement in energy, emotions, and pain levels, compared with 18 per cent of the controls. After treatment, red cell magnesium was normal in all of those who received magnesium, but only in one of the 17 controls.

Those who improved with magnesium need to be monitored to see how long the benefit lasts, and how often the treatment should be given. The results of this important study are encouraging, and hopefully the trial will be repeated to confirm the role of magnesium. Many sufferers have already found some benefit from taking magnesium by mouth, but it is more effective when given by injection. The treatment is safe, so long as injection into a vein is avoided. At the time of writing, it is suggested that patients have their red cell magnesium level tested first before having a course of injections.

In M.E., there is a delay in recovery of muscle fibres after contracting, and a low level of magnesium in the cell may contribute to this.

If you supplement magnesium by mouth, take enough to give about 500 mg elemental magnesium a day, until there is improvement. Then about 300 mg daily as maintenance, depending on your symptoms of muscle weakness, twitchings, or mental symptoms such as panic attacks and insomnia. Amino acid chelated magnesium is a good form to take.

Some doctors advise that calcium should be taken as well, as a separate supplement, about 500 mg a day.

Selenium

This mineral occurs widely in food, and its functions are not yet fully understood. The important role of selenium which *has* been researched is as an anti-oxidant, mopping up free radicals, and thus it helps protect cells from damage, ageing, and cancerous changes.

The relevance of selenium to M.E. is that sometimes severe chemical sensitivity develops, and it is thought that free radicals plus chemical molecules can further impair cell membranes, and contribute to muscle weakness and mental dysfunction. (This may explain why it is not uncommon for a patient to find that he or she has greater muscle power when in an unpolluted area, but collapses in a narrow street full of petrol fumes.)

Many M.E. patients with chemical sensitivities have improved on a regime which includes all the anti-oxidants (vitamins A, C, and E, and selenium). However, selenium is toxic in high doses, and a supplement should not exceed 200 mcg a day.

Essential Fatty Acid Supplements

The role of EFAs is discussed in Chapter 11. If one is having pure vegetable oils, vegetables, nuts, and fish in a good diet, why is there any need for supplements?

Linoleic acid in food is converted to prostaglandin E1 (which is anti-inflammatory and boosts white cell function), via gamma linolenic acid on the pathway (see page 148).

The conversion of linoleic acid to GLA can be blocked by several things, including viral infections. Taking GLA in evening primrose oil by-passes this block, and the GLA can go on to form the helpful prostaglandin E1.

EFAs and their products are needed to make cell membranes, and are important constituents of white matter in nervous tissue. EFA supplements are used with success to help patients who have Multiple Sclerosis. MS is a disease of myelin tissue, but defects in cell membranes have been discovered, and present evidence suggests that the underlying problem is an inability to handle fats properly. An initial virus infection may be implicated.

Professor P. O. Behan and colleagues at Glasgow

carried out a double-blind trial of EFAs on post-viral syndrome (Behan, 1990). 63 patients received either *Efamol Marine* (8 × 500 mg a day) or a similar looking placebo (liquid paraffin) for three months. After three months, 85 per cent of the patients receiving EFAs and 17 per cent of those on the placebo noted overall improvement, and the level of improvement was much greater in the treated group. In the treated patients, blood levels of EFAs which had been abnormal before the trial returned to normal.

What seems clear is that not only is EFA supplementation advisable for M.E., but that high doses are needed, at least 3 gm per day. The Glasgow trial used *Efamol Marine*, which contains fish oil as well as evening primrose oil. Although there has been no tested comparison between the effectiveness of evening primrose oil alone, or combined with fish oil, anecdotal evidence suggests that the combination of GLA (in evening primrose oil, and also in borage oil) with fish oil is best.

EFAs need adequate zinc, magnesium, and vitamins B_6, C, and E to work properly.

Amino Acids

Amino acids are the basic building blocks for the manufacture of all proteins in the body, including antibodies, all the lymphokines produced by white cells, digestive enzymes, neuro-transmitters and hormones. Without these building blocks, taking vitamin and mineral supplements may be a waste of money. Certain amino acids are known to be needed for proper brain function, and the amino acids *tryptophan* and *phenylalanine* can improve mood.

Unless you can have a full analysis of your amino acid levels carried out, you will not know which, if any, you are short of. Anyone with M.E. who has symptoms that suggest poor absorption together with depression is advised to try taking a supplement of 'free-form amino acids'. These are available either on prescription or as capsules in most health food shops, and should be taken between meals with some water three times a day.

I know of a number of M.E. people who did not improve with a very nutritious diet, plus supplements, but felt an increase in strength and clearing of the mind after starting to take free-form amino acids – myself included.

Summary of Supplements

Ideally, someone considering taking nutritional supplements should consult a physician or biochemist who specializes in nutrition, and have his or her individual nutritional needs worked out. This is not usually possible, due to distances and the cost of a consultation and tests. Failing the opportunity for such advice, then suitable supplements for someone with M.E. would be:

- A good quality multivitamin and mineral tablet daily – ideally one with high levels of B vitamins, and which is yeast-free.
- Evening primrose oil (or equivalent): 3 gm daily
- Zinc: 20–50 mg, at night
- Magnesium: 200–300 mg daily
- Selenium: 100 mcg daily
- Vitamin E: 100–200 I.U. daily
- Calcium Pantothenate: 300 mg daily (up to 1,000 mg a day if very stressed or if badly allergic)
- Vitamin C: minimum 1–3 gm a day, more if very unwell or exposed to infection.
- If indicated, amino acids, pancreatic enzymes, or hydrochloric acid.

There will be no benefit in exceeding these doses without medical supervision. There may be ill effects from overdosing, and certainly loss of money. Most will be excreted from the body if taken in excess.

Suggested Further Reading

Earl Mindell, *The Vitamin Bible*, (Arlington Books, 1985).

Linus Pauling, *How to Live Longer and Feel Better*, (W.H. Freeman, 1986).

Judy Graham, *Evening Primrose Oil*, (Thorsons, 1989).

Robert Erdmann and Meirion Jones, *The Amino Revolution*, (Century, 1988).

Chapter 13

Candida Albicans

Possibly two-thirds of M.E. sufferers have their condition made worse by an infection with the yeast called Candida. This is a controversial subject, and there are widely differing opinions within orthodox and alternative medical professions. At one extreme are people who claim that Candida is the No. 1 culprit in all M.E. patients, and that if you can get rid of it you will be a great deal better, or even cured. At the other end are those who cannot accept that Candida infection has anything whatsoever to do with M.E., or indeed any ill health, and who feel trying to treat it is a waste of time.

A lot of people have now heard the word Candida, but for those who have not, Candida Albicans is one of the many bugs which is to be found living in and on all of us. It is a fungus, one of the yeast family of organisms, and is best known for causing thrush in the mouths of babies – sore white, moist plaques in the mouth and on the tongue, and thrush in the vaginas of women (which is where the babies pick it up, during birth). It can also cause nappy rash, and soreness and itching around the anus and genitals in adults.

This yeast lives in small numbers in the gut, and on the skin, especially in warm moist areas. In a healthy person with a strong defence system, Candida keeps its place and does not cause any symptoms. It is so prevalent that at least 90 per cent of children have had exposure to it by the time they are six months old (based on tests done on skin reactions).

The most extreme cases of Candida infection in all parts of the body (including the bloodstream, lungs and brain) are in ill people with severely collapsed immunity. These include some leukaemia sufferers, people on immuno-suppressive treatment, those with overwhelming infections which wipe out the bone marrow, or those with advanced AIDS.

It must be emphasized again that the mild immune dysfunction in the M.E. syndrome is *quite different* to the immune failure seen in the above examples.

Candida is only one of a huge variety of yeasts, viruses and bacteria which live on, in and around us. The large bowel contains several pounds in weight of bacteria, most of which are necessary for the manufacture of some vitamins, the fermentation of undigested food, and the breakdown of mucus. They stay in their place because of the colon wall and the body's efficient immune surveillance system.

There are some circumstances which may allow Candida to multiply and cause trouble:

Factors that Favour Candida Overgrowth

- Warmth and moisture
- Sugar – e.g. in diabetes, excess sugar in diet. (Bread rises with yeast and sugar, and sugar is needed to ferment alcoholic drinks).
- A weakened defence system
- Altered hormone levels – such as are caused by the contraceptive pill, pregnancy, steroid drugs (cortisone, prednisolone).
- Taking broad-spectrum antibiotics – because these not only kill off the bugs that are making you ill, but also destroy large numbers of the friendly bacteria that exist in the colon.

The fact that broad-spectrum antibiotics kill off significant numbers of friendly bacteria leads to a relative 'overgrowth' of yeasts which are left unharmed by antibiotics. The imbalance of microbes thus created is known as *dysbiosis* – a disharmony of bugs.

Dysbiosis may contribute to many conditions of ill health, including M.E. Although unknown by many doctors, dysbiosis is recognized and treated by veterinarians. Antibiotics used for a short course, and selected to kill specific bugs, such as penicillin for tonsillitis, do less harm. It is the broad-spectrum antibiotics, designed to 'kill all known germs', that cause dysbiosis, especially if given repeatedly or over a period of time.

Two conditions for which long-term broad-spectrum antibiotics tend to be prescribed are acne and recurrent cystitis. It is unfortunate that these problems may actually be caused by a Candida infection, and made worse by antibiotics.

Another source of long-term antibiotics may be from meat and poultry that comes from intensively-reared animals. Their foodstuff may have antibiotics added to prevent infections that result from poor, overcrowded conditions. The quantity is of course small, but must have some effect on humans over a period of time.

Let us not ignore the fact that antibiotics have saved thousands of lives. Pneumonia used to kill many people, and infection and gangrene killed many thousands in the First World War. In the last two decades there has been a tendency to overprescribe broad-spectrum antibiotics, however, often using them as an umbrella tactic, instead of encouraging the body to overcome what may be quite a minor infection, or for a virus infection which is not touched by antibiotics anyway. So a generation has grown up who may have had antibiotics many times in childhood for ear or throat infections, in adolescence for spots, and as young adults for bouts of flu or bladder infections.

Given favourable conditions, Candida can proliferate quite fast, and cause local symptoms:

• vaginal thrush
• cystitis

- infection of prostate gland and male genitals
- skin rashes of the groin or armpits
- fungal infections of the nails
- white patches and ulcers on the gums and mouth
- infection of tongue, throat and gullet

These are all surface infections.

It is thought that Candida may produce toxins by its action on fermenting sugar, producing a nasty substance called *Acetaldehyde*. This would explain why the symptoms of a bowel Candida infection can resemble those of an alcoholic hangover, i.e. headache, nausea, lack of concentration, irritability, and a general feeling of having been poisoned.

The ability of Candida to ferment sugar is the basis of the sugar fermentation test used in investigations of the gut.

Candida may possibly contribute to many conditions, including cystitis, prostatitis, endometriosis, irritable bowel syndrome, vaginal discharge, premenstrual tension, rapid mood changes, sudden weight gain, joint pains, muscle aching, fatigue, athlete's foot, acne, sneezing, asthma, food allergies, chemical allergies, abdominal bloating, and loss of sexual drive.

These symptoms may result not from the yeast infection itself, but from hypersensitivity to Candida Albicans.

As you can see, much of this list overlaps with typical M.E. symptoms. However, there are some clear indications of Candida overgrowth or hypersensitivity.

Candida Assessment Guide

History

- Have you been on oral contraceptives for a year or more?
- Have you ever had steroids (prednisolone, cortisone)?

- Have you had frequent courses of antibiotics, or a course lasting six weeks or more?
- Have you had long-term antibiotics for acne?
- Have you been pregnant?
- Have you had immuno-suppressant drugs?

Symptoms

- Have you had cystitis, vaginitis, or prostatitis?
- Have you had thrush more than once?
- Have you ever had fungal infection of nails or skin, e.g. athlete's foot?
- Do you have chemical allergies – worse from exposure to tobacco smoke, petrol, perfumes, paints, etc.?
- Are your symptoms worse in damp weather or in a damp and mouldy house?
- Do you have premenstrual bloating, irritability, or rapid mood swings?
- Do you have bloating after meals, or alternating diarrhoea and constipation?
- Are the symptoms worse for eating sweet foods, or alcohol?
- Do you crave sweets, or alcohol?
- Do you have an itching or burning sensation in the anus?

If you answer *yes* to one or more of the history questions, and have two or more positive symptoms, then it is likely that Candida plays some part in your illness. However, *Candida does not cause M.E.*, it is just one of the possible complications. 'Chronic mucocutaneous candidiasis is a common complication in immunodeficiency affecting T lymphocytes' (Matthews, 1988).

There is no one reliable blood test that can tell you if Candida Albicans is causing your symptoms. However, the combination of finding antibodies to Candida, together with changes in T lymphocytes in the blood, have been found in most patients with obvious Candida-related illness in a study in the USA. Skin testing with diluted Candida extract produces a positive result in most of the population, so this test does not help. Candida can be isolated from the gut of everyone, if it is looked for. The best test at present is to treat it and see if symptoms improve.

It is quite possible to have a Candida problem without having the obvious symptoms, such as thrush. Chemical sensitivity and an intolerance to some foods are extremely common. The headaches, irritability, lethargy and lack of concentration that are so common in M.E. may result from:

a) the virus interfering with brain cells
b) toxins such as acetaldehyde, produced by Candida
c) chemical sensitivity
d) absorption of larger than usual molecules of partly digested food, particularly proteins.

Before studying ways of overcoming Candida infections, please understand that:

a) not everyone with M.E. has a Candida problem, although probably at least two-thirds are affected; this figure is based on a questionnaire study, and is probably an underestimate.
b) treating Candida effectively will make you feel better if there is a problem, and may well clear up or improve the allergies. You will not cure M.E. immediately. However, through removing one of the stresses on the immune system the body's natural healing powers will have a better chance of fighting M.E.
c) if you are going to embark on an anti-Candida programme, it is worth giving it a serious trial for at least three months, rather than doing it half-heartedly and then deciding it doesn't work.

There are three parts to the attack on Candida:

1. modifying the diet to starve it of sugar

2. strengthening the body's natural resistance with nutritional supplements
3. taking specific anti-Candida medication.

The Anti-Candida Diet

The reasons for making changes in how you eat are to deprive Candida of its nourishment, which is sugar, to avoid consuming any other moulds or fungi, and to eat nutritiously to strengthen the natural defences.

Now, if you have put into practice the guidelines for healthy eating described in Chapter 11, then you are half way there. A *strict* anti-Candida diet would also prohibit bread made with yeast, cheese, vinegar, anything else fermented such as soy sauce; it would also restrict carbohydrate intake to about 80 gm a day, and would prohibit milk and its products. What is more important than restricting carbohydrates is to cut out all refined carbohydrates – sugar of all kinds and refined flour, and to eat more complex carbohydrates.

If an M.E. patient is already underweight, he or she must *not* embark on a diet which is going to make him or her lose even more. It is just as important to feed the patient as to starve the Candida.

A strict regime also advises no fruit. In practice, a sensible compromise is to have no more than one piece of fresh fruit a day, and to avoid those high in sugar (honeydew melon, bananas) and those with yeasts on the skin (grapes).

Foods Allowed

Potatoes
Fresh vegetables of all kinds, especially garlic, onion and
    members of the cabbage family
Meat, fish, eggs – preferably antibiotic and hormone-
    free
Wholegrains – brown rice, oats, muesli (no sugar),
    crispbreads, oatcakes, wholemeal pasta

Pure vegetable oils
Freshly shelled nuts
Pulses – lentils, beans, soya (but caution if these products give you gas, and they must be well-cooked)
Water, tea, fresh fruit juice, such as squeezed orange

Foods to Avoid

Sugar of all kinds – including molasses, honey, and brown sugar
Anything containing sugar – read labels
Alcohol in all forms – it makes M.E. and Candida patients ill
Fermented food and drink – vinegar, ginger ale, soy sauce, tofu, miso, tempeh (all soya derivatives), buttermilk, cheeses – especially blue cheese
Ready shelled nuts and dried fruit. These often have moulds on the surface, and dried fruit is rich in fruit sugar
Melon and grapes
Mushrooms and truffles
Fruit juices, unless freshly squeezed
Anything pickled
Any food which is mouldy, so vegetables and fruit should be as fresh as possible

Foods Allowed in Moderation

Wholemeal bread – ideally none at all if made with yeast for the first four weeks, then perhaps two medium-sized slices a day if tolerated (if not, it will probably cause bloating and worsening of symptoms)
Milk, live, unsweetened yoghourt
Cottage cheese
Fresh fruit

On a really strict diet, you would not have anything from this final category, nor any milk or milk products. It is thought that the lactose in milk helps feed Candida. If you feel you want to try the strict diet for the first four weeks or so, that is fine, provided you eat enough overall, and do not find the whole exercise too stressful. A lot depends on how you have been eating up till now, your weight, and also your motivation.

The most important things to avoid are: *sugar, alcohol and fermented foods*.

Until recently, the standard advice given was to avoid eating anything containing yeast, moulds or fungi. Dr William G. Crook, in his book *The Yeast Connection*, believes that not all Candida patients are affected by other yeasts. He suggests that one should cut out all yeast-containing foods for at least a week, then test to see if yeast causes trouble. This can be done by chewing a fragment of brewer's yeast tablet. If no symptoms develop after 10 minutes, continue to have pieces of yeast tablet for an hour, then a whole tablet if there is no reaction. Then try some food such as mushrooms the next day. Of course, if there is any reaction early on in the testing, you should stop and either assume you have a yeast sensitivity, or try again a few days later.

The point of finding out if other yeasts and moulds affect you is that if they do not, then you can eat ordinary bread. Dr Crook advises that even if one is not yeast sensitive, a person trying to deal with Candida should still be moderate in having yeasts and moulds in his or her diet, and should stop them and retest if the condition gets worse.

Another great benefit from finding you are not affected by yeasts is that you can take brewer's yeast tablets as Vitamin B supplements; they are also the best source of Chromium, a mineral which is essential for proper blood-sugar control.

However, alcohol should still be avoided, whether or not yeasts upset you.

A person who already enjoys healthy eating will find the anti-Candida changes easier.

Supplements

Probiotics

Unlike antibiotics, probiotics replenish the families of friendly bugs living in the colon, and therefore they restore normal balance and help displace Candida.

There are various preparations on the market, the most effective being a mixture of *Lactobacillus acidophilus* and *Bifidobacteria*. L. acidophilus occurs in some yoghourt cultures, and can be bought in capsule, powder or tablet form. Yoghourt, to be of any use, must be live, not pasteurized.

Probiotics should be taken between meals, one capsule or ¼ teaspoon of powder (or as instructed) three times a day. The L. acidophilus and Bifidobacteriae should multiply in the large bowel and gradually build up numbers there.

Another way to take probiotics is to start your own yoghourt culture, using some of the organisms from the marketed probiotic preparations. This produces a yoghourt with a more powerful brand of the correct bugs than most ready-made brands. Even people who are lactose intolerant can usually cope with yoghourt, because the lactobacilli and other bugs eat the lactose while they are turning the milk into yoghourt. The longest-living peoples of the world, found around the Black Sea, reputedly eat a lot of yoghourt.

Other Supplements to Help Fight Candida

Those suggested in Chapter 12 are ideal.

Magnesium seems to be important for people with Candida infection. For some reason it does not appear to be absorbed, or else is lost to the system. At least 300 mg daily should be aimed at, and make sure you are getting vitamin B_6 in your daily pills.

Also especially helpful against Candida are:

• Biotin – 300 mcg, taken with acidophilus

- Garlic – fresh, as much as you can stand; use the flesh and juice immediately after crushing, in salad dressing or mixed with any food; if left it deteriorates and develops an unpleasant smell. The best bought garlic comes in freeze-dried enteric coated capsules, from health food shops. Garlic perles are less effective, as much of the antifungal part has been removed in the processing.
- Cold-pressed olive oil – about a tablespoon daily, such as on salads. It is the oleic acid which has natural antifungal properties. Perhaps this is why a lot of M.E. and Candida symptoms seem to improve during a holiday in Greece, Italy or Spain?

Antifungal Treatments

Nystatin

Nystatin and fungilin (see below) are the most commonly used agents to kill Candida. There is little point in having treatment with nystatin without employing dietary means, however, because if the conditions in which Candida flourished are not altered, then the symptoms will just keep recurring. This is borne out by thousands of women with recurrent thrush, who have many repeated prescriptions of nystatin or other pessaries, but no advice about changing the body environment to discourage Candida – so, naturally, all the nystatin does is to suppress the problem temporarily.

Nystatin comes in tablets, suspension (for babies and children), vaginal pessaries, and powder. For treating general symptoms of Candida overgrowth, the powder preparation seems to work better than the tablets.

Because the start of treatment frequently brings on more severe symptoms, due to a 'die-off' reaction from dead and burst yeast cells, *it is essential to start with small doses.*

It is also best to start by starving Candida of sugar, so have at least two weeks on the anti-Candida diet, probiotics and supplements before starting on nystatin or fungilin.

Dosage

Start with one tablet or ⅛ teaspoon of nystatin a day. Each of these has 500,000 units of nystatin.

After two days increase to twice daily, and after another two days to four times daily – i.e. a total of four tablets or ½ teaspoon of powder per day.

The powder does not dissolve well in water, but a good way to mix it is to put the day's total dose in a small bottle, such as an empty vitamin container, add water, and shake vigorously with the top screwed on. Then divide this mixture into two or more lots, and mix each lot with more water. This saves further mixing and stirring, and you'll know you have taken the day's quota.

After two or three days, you may feel much worse. All the worst symptoms may be magnified, and you may feel quite awful – abdominal pains, sweating, headache, rapid pulse, insomnia, crying, etc. *Do not give up!* These signs mean that Candida yeast spores are bursting and dying, and releasing their toxins into your system.

Drink lots of water, take extra vitamin C, and carry on with the nystatin. After a further few days it will all get much better. If the reaction is really unbearable, go on with the nystatin but in a tiny dose for a few days, then start gradually building up again.

Nystatin has a nasty taste. If you cannot bear it, a little diluted fresh fruit juice in the mixture is permissible. The maximum dose of nystatin tolerated may be up to 4 million units daily, i.e. 8 tablets of ½ million each, or 1 teaspoon (heaped) of powder.

Powder or Tablets?

Tablets are much easier to take, help you avoid the

unpleasant taste, and are more readily obtainable on prescription in the UK.

However, powder reaches parts that tablets don't: Candida lurks in the mouth, between the teeth, and in the throat, nose, and gullet. If you can obtain powder *and* tablets, then a good compromise is to take powder when at home and tablets if you go out or are away from home. When you take powder mixed up with water, keep the first mouthful in your mouth and swill it around for a few seconds before swallowing. This will get the nystatin into the 'cracks and crevices'. You can gargle with it as well, especially if you have a sore throat, which may be due to Candida as well as a virus.

Fungilin (Amphotericin B)

This comes as lozenges, which are good to suck or chew to clear the fungus from the mouth and throat, but their dosage is too low to be effective in the gut.

As 100 mg tablets, fungilin is taken in a dose of one or two tablets four times a day. Similar 'die-off' symptoms may occur as with nystatin, and mean the treatment needs to be continued.

There does not seem to be any hard evidence on whether nystatin or fungilin work best, but fungilin is thought to penetrate the bowel wall more effectively. Both are well-tolerated, are not absorbed from the gut, and are effective against Candida. Fungilin is usually better tolerated than nystatin, however, as nystatin may cause side-effects such as nausea after a time.

Ketoconazole (Nizoral)

This antifungal drug is absorbed into the bloodstream, and is very effective. However it may cause liver damage, and patients require regular liver function tests while taking it.

Fluconazole (Diflucan)

This is a relatively new drug, and so far seems to be both

effective and safe. However, it is expensive, and may not be easy to obtain in the UK on NHS prescription unless other antifungal drugs prove ineffective.

Some research of interest – in the USA, Dr Carol Jessop (University of California, 1990) monitored 1200 patients over five years for their response to antifungal ketoconazole treatment. The results 'suggest that colonization of yeast may play a role in aetiology of Chronic Fatigue Syndrome, and also suggests that patients may benefit from systemic anti-yeast therapy and a decrease of sugars in the diet.'

It was noted that 85 per cent of the patients in the trial had been treated with the antibiotic tetracycline for two or more years in the past.

Probiotics should be continued along with the antifungal drugs.

It may be necessary to treat Candida in various other situations with different methods. Nystatin and fungilin can be used as lozenges, to treat the mouth, throat and gullet; pessaries to treat vaginal infections; and creams for the skin.

If large doses by mouth are not clearing the mental and gut symptoms, it may be worth administering nystatin directly to the lower bowel via an enema, or even by using the pessaries as suppositories. This is best done by clearing the lower bowel with an ordinary enema, then giving a small retention enema of warm water containing ¼ teaspoon of nystatin powder, or a crushed tablet of fungilin or nystatin. This is not an easy task for someone who is ill and weak, so unless a nurse or a helper who is trained to give enemas is at hand, this idea may not be practical.

Treatment of Candida may have to be continued for a year or more, and, according to progress, the antifungal agent can be cut down or stopped, and then the diet can be relaxed. However, vigilance needs to be maintained. Having got better, do *not* start having sugar, alcohol and cakes – you will certainly get the Candida back!

Colon Cleansing by Fibre

Some therapists advise adding special fibres, such as oat bran fibre or psyllium husks, to a diet high in vegetables. This helps remove old, sticky, putrefying matter from the lining of the colon. You must drink a lot of water if you take psyllium husks, however: otherwise there is a small risk of intestinal obstruction. A preparation of linseeds, e.g. *Linusit*, is safer than psyllium, and is recommended.

Colonic Washouts

Washing out the large bowel by a sort of high-level enema, using warm water, was fashionable at the beginning of this century. A few people who suffer from constipation, possibly Candida overgrowth, or possibly M.E., have reported an improvement in symptoms after a course of this treatment. However, there is no evidence to show that colonic irrigation produces any lasting benefit to M.E. patients; it may even be counterproductive, as the procedure washes out essential minerals, may damage the lining of the bowel, and can bring on a severe relapse. It is an expensive therapy, and is *not* recommended for people who are ill with M.E. Constipation should be treated by less drastic means, such as diet change, vitamin C, extra fibre, and mild aperients.

Capristatin

Some fatty acids have been shown to destroy fungi. One such is caprylic acid, which is derived from coconuts. It is effective if taken as a slow release preparation, called *capristatin*, which reaches the large bowel before it is absorbed. Capristatin may be very useful for anyone who cannot tolerate nystatin or fungilin, but is not obtainable on prescription. (See Appendix A for supplier.)

Antifungal Foods

As previously mentioned, garlic, onion, and vegetables

of the cabbage family (*Brassicas*) all have antifungal qualities due to the sulphur-containing chemicals in them. They should all be eaten liberally, as well as olive oil, for its oleic acid content.

Herbs

A tea made from a tree bark (Taheebo tree, also known as Pau d'Arco) has antifungal and immune system-enhancing effects.

Aloe Vera is a plant with antifungal properties. It is available in cream, ointment, or lotion for external use, and also as a preparation to drink.

Summary

If you decide to have a go at getting rid of Candida, you should first change your diet and take probiotics and nutritional supplements; then after a month or so consider having long-term anti-Candida therapy. Some people can control their Candida by diet and probiotics alone.

If you have a definite lessening of your symptoms, then do keep on with the programme for at least six months. If there is no improvement after two months on the diet and antifungals, then you can say you have given it a fair trial and leave it. Many people who maintain that treating Candida did not help them have not done the programme seriously and consistently.

Case History

The following story is typical of someone with a Candida illness:

Mrs C. A., aged 44 (20 at onset).

Mrs A. started her illness with a bad attack of flu when she was 20, then had two bad bouts of gastroenteritis. At the time, she suffered from a bad marriage and overwork, lived in a damp house, and had recently had a breast lump removed.

'After the illness started, in 1968, with a bad dose of flu, I had constant diarrhoea and a sore throat. My joints went haywire at the same time, I had pins and needles in my hands and feet, severe abdominal pain and wind, and was very tired. My personality changed, with a short temper and irritability. I felt awful most of the time. In 1969 we moved, and I found I was getting tonsillitis again and again. Because of family trouble I saw a psychiatrist. *All the antibiotics I had gave me fungus in the mouth, so I was given nystatin to suck.*

'I remember craving sweet things, perspiring a lot, and getting trembly if I didn't eat. I was drinking two litres of Coke a day!

'In 1972 we moved again. I worked full-time, still felt awful. My knees suddenly went, with dreadful pains. The hospital said it was probably "arthritis caused by a virus". I also had eczema (since three years before this). I became allergic to many things – *all* painkillers brought me out in big lumps, and I'd have difficulty breathing. Red wine made me short of breath, but it wasn't until 1985 that I found out all the foods I was allergic to.

'I am now getting better, but my symptoms were: dreadful fatigue; any exercise made me feel drunk, or would give me migraine and make me unable to walk straight (felt drunk) the next day; joint pains, muscle pains, PMT, blurred vision, feeling very cold, sweating, tinnitus, wind, bloating and diarrhoea, chest pains, difficulty breathing, and allergies. At present, improved, I can walk slowly for about half an hour, but feel whacked afterwards. If I rest before I have exhausted myself, I feel better and can avoid the headaches.

'I started to feel better seven or eight years ago. I had remarried to a good man and felt content. Then I tried to make myself fit – jogging, aerobics, tennis – I pushed myself, then started to go downhill. I also started a full-time degree course. After a year, the throat problems came back, then the chest infection, and after that back came the tiredness, joint pains, blurred vision, etc.

'I am now seeing a doctor at an Allergy Clinic. I am on a strict diet of vegetables, eggs, fish, meat, herb tea, garlic, onions, oils, and psyllium husks. I eat no fruit yet, also no dairy products. I take acidophilus and vitamins. I have had no sore throat for months, the eczema has gone, and there is general improvement. I rest as well.'

'As a child I had blood-poisoning several times from insect bites or little cuts.

'By age 19, I had had four pregnancies, developing an inflammation of the womb after the second of these, which caused me wind and bloating of the stomach from then on. I'd had athlete's foot all through childhood, lots of mouth ulcers, fungus disease of the skin when I was 16, and a fungus infection in the stitches given me after my first baby was born.

'I used to eat yeast with sugar as a snack, also eggs whipped up with sugar. I liked blue cheeses, pickles, and lots of Coke – my diet was very poor'.

Comment

All the signs of fungus infestation right from her teens, yet no doctor spotted it. This story shows that M.E. and Candida symptoms overlap. In her case, chronic yeast infection became much worse aged 20, following the virus infection. Is her diagnosis M.E., or chronic Candida? She probably has both.

She had a poor natural resistance to infection from childhood – the 'stage was set' to develop M.E. syndrome. Multiple allergies are frequently present with a yeast infection.

Suggested Further Reading

William G. Crook MD, *The Yeast Connection* (Future Health, 1984).
Leon Chaitow, *Candida Albicans* (Thorsons, 1991).

Chapter 14

Allergies

The word allergy comes from two Greek words, *allos* meaning other, *ergon* meaning energy.

An allergy is an altered reaction to some outside stimulus. Something that provokes such an altered reaction is called an *allergen*.

Another word for an allergic reaction could be hypersensitivity. An allergic response is one that is different from the response of the majority of people. Most people can breathe in grass pollens, only a minority develop hay fever. Most people can happily eat oranges, a few people react to them. The allergies that are easily recognized are: hay fever, asthma, eczema, migraine, skin reactions such as nettle rash, and collapse after bee stings.

Hypersensitive reactions also occur to inhaled chemicals, to traces of chemicals in food and water, or even to apparently harmless common foods. The understanding of different types of allergy has broadened considerably in the last 40 years, the pioneers of observation and research of food and chemical allergies being Dr Albert Rowe in the 1920s, and Dr Theron G. Randolph and his colleagues in the USA in the 1950s.

Estimates of the numbers of people with M.E. who have allergies vary from 20 per cent to 70 per cent.

One explanation is that the immune system's defences initially act against infection, but do not switch off, because the virus becomes persistent. (See immune activation, page 54). The body's defences thus become overreactive to other foreign substances as well as to the virus.

There is a difference between food allergy and food intolerance. A true food allergy is usually fixed, and may be inherited. The reaction happens very quickly, and even the tiniest amount of the food may provoke a severe response. Symptoms could be asthma, swelling of the face, 'nettle rash', or collapse with vomiting. Food intolerance is less easy to diagnose, as symptoms may not develop for up to 24 hours, and a reaction may depend on the amount eaten. Intolerance to commonly eaten foods may come and go, and if a culprit food is avoided for some weeks, the intolerance may disappear.

Most apparent food 'allergy' in M.E. is in fact food intolerance; however since food allergy is the recognized word, it will be used in this chapter. Not everyone who has multiple allergies has M.E., but in many there is an underlying Candida condition.

Allergens are of three types:

1. Those ingested – foods, liquids, chemicals in food
2. Those inhaled – pollen, house dust mite, moulds, animal fur, chemicals (formaldehyde, petrol, alcohol, aerosols, smoke)
3. Those one comes in contact with – metals (nickel in bra and suspenders) rings, watches; dyes; various chemicals

Recent research by Dr Hunter at Cambridge (Hunter, 1991) has suggested that many cases of food intolerance may be due to the presence of abnormal gut flora plus a lower activity of certain gut enzymes. 'Specific food residues are broken down by colonic microflora with the production of chemicals, which in susceptible people with low concentrations of liver enzymes, pass into the circulation to produce distant symptoms.' This is supported by the finding of abnormal colonic bacteria in other diseases – e.g. rheumatoid arthritis, irritable bowel syndrome (see dysbiosis, page 172).

The successful management of allergies is not only to remove the allergens, but to help the immune system to recover. The practical problems arise when a patient is found to be reacting badly to so many things that avoiding them all causes malnutrition, and total isolation from the world. For this reason, very restricted diets in M.E. do more harm than good, and can lead to malnutrition and worsening of the M.E..

Many M.E. symptoms are the same as those resulting from allergic reactions. Signs suggestive of allergies are:

- Symptoms worse after food, such as rapid pulse, wheezing, abdominal pains, bloating, sudden feeling of cold, headache, joint pain, sudden mood change, sweating
- Symptoms improve on fasting
- Feeling worse when in traffic jams, in city centres, on exposure to aerosol spray, fresh paint, etc., suggesting chemical allergies
- Feeling better for being outside in the fresh air, maybe because of indoor air chemical pollution
- Sneezing and itchy eyes – hay fever
- Symptoms improve on change of location

Allergic symptoms are so numerous that there is no point making a list of them. It is the variability of symptoms on exposure to different foods and chemicals that is typical of allergy. If you suspect that food allergies are causing some of your problems, then adding details of what you eat and drink to your diary, or keeping a separate food diary, may help to pin-point culprit foods.

However, there may be foods which you eat every day that are making you ill. Instead of an acute reaction to something rarely eaten, such as swelling and itching after strawberries, you can be chronically unwell by eating something so regularly that it never gets cleared from the system. This is called a *masked allergy*, and is also a form of addiction.

What happens is that repeated exposure to the food leads to general ill health due to the constant stress on the immune system (see stress adaptation page 114).

Avoidance of the allergen for 24 hours or more may lead to withdrawal symptoms, as happens when an alcoholic dries out, or a cigarette smoker stops smoking. These withdrawal symptoms settle down in a few days, then the subject becomes extra-sensitive to the allergen and re-exposure causes more dramatic symptoms than when it was being taken every day – when the reaction was being *masked* through partial adaptation to the substance.

The elimination and provocation-testing method of food allergy detection is based on understanding this masked allergy phenomenon. If you avoid the suspect allergen, allow it to disappear from your gut (which takes up to five days), and then eat it again, it will cause the symptoms to reappear more strongly. If there are no ill effects, then it is regarded as safe.

The same principle applies to a chemical masked allergy. For example, a woman with chronic headaches, depression and fatigue went on holiday to a small Mediterranean island, and after three days she felt wonderful. On returning home to her kitchen, which had a gas cooker, she felt absolutely dreadful; her depression and headache returned with a vengeance within a few hours of entering the house. Fortunately, the departure to a place of clean air had also sharpened her senses, so that on entering the kitchen she detected a slight smell of gas. After the gas appliance was removed her symptoms cleared up.

The mechanism causing symptoms from exposure to allergens is complex. Frequently it is several allergens combined, plus other stresses, which produce symptoms.

A good model for understanding this phenomenon is to think of it as a barrel of water. If the level of water is too high it overflows, just as, if the level of the sum total of stresses is too high, one further exposure to an allergen produces a reaction.

The final drop of water into the barrel is like the last

straw that broke the camel's back. It is the sum total of all stresses that causes symptoms. So then, if one can lower the level of water in the barrel, a further measure of water may be all right and not cause symptoms.

Therefore, symptoms may improve somewhat if the total of stresses on the immune system is lowered. Often the last straw is not an allergen, but a psychological stress. For example, a child with eczema very possibly has a cow's milk intolerance, masked because it is drunk daily; the child dutifully drinks the milk and is chronically miserable and itching. When he or she goes to a new school, or has a row in the classroom, the eczema flares up very badly. Is the mental stress to blame, or the cow's milk? The answer is both, of course. But if the cow's milk is removed, probably the school stress will have less of an effect on the eczema.

It is quite unrealistic for M.E. patients to try and avoid every single thing they react to, and there is some cause for concern if someone who is already ill starves him- or herself on a strict elimination diet. Therefore, much of the management of allergies may rest in compromise.

Let us look at the various stresses and allergens that may be filling up the water barrel:

Physical exercise
Mental stress
Airborne allergens – house dust mite, pet hairs, pollens
Electromagnetic stress – TV, VDUs, electric cables
Chemical allergens – traffic fumes, aerosols, gas leaks,
    fresh paint, perfumes, new carpets, printing ink, etc.
Food intolerances – e.g. to wheat, milk, egg, pork
Some ongoing infection

Some of these things you cannot do anything about. What you *should* do is avoid as many of them as you can.

Detecting Allergies

None of these testing methods is 100 per cent accurate,

and in a very sensitive person, allergies can change from day to day. However, the most important sensitivities come up repeatedly on subsequent testing, and these are the ones that the patient needs to avoid. The best – also the cheapest – way to test for foods that cause problems is by an elimination diet.

The Elimination, Unmasking and Challenge Diet

There are various ways of detecting food allergies.

The elimination, unmasking and challenge diet is the simplest and probably most accurate method of diagnosing food allergy. The disadvantage is that it is time-consuming. *It should not be undertaken without medical supervision by any child, nor by any patient suffering from depression, epilepsy, or asthma,* because of the possibly dangerous consequence of a severe reaction on food testing after avoidance.

The patient fasts for five days, drinking only spring water, or else eating a few foods which are rarely eaten. Two foods are usually used, for example lamb and pears, or cod and broccoli. During the fast, any symptoms are noted, as well as any cravings for particular foods. If it is not a complete fast, it should be continued for at least a week, to allow symptoms time to clear up. If all the pre-fast symptoms are still there after a week, either food allergy was not responsible, or one of the few foods used was not safe.

Foods are then reintroduced one at a time, one each day, the less commonly eaten foods first. If there is a reaction on testing, it usually happens within 24 hours, although it may be delayed for 48 hours. All symptoms are noted, including the resting pulse rate before and up to two hours after a test food is eaten. A food that produces no reaction can be reintroduced, and as testing proceeds the patient hopefully develops a gradually wider range of safe foodstuffs.

However, this method requires strong motivation and meticulousness on the part of the patient, and sometimes a delayed reaction may confuse the picture.

The Stone Age Diet

This is a modified elimination diet. It was first used in Britain for allergy testing and treatment by Dr Richard Mackarness, a psychiatrist at Basingstoke.

Our hunter-gatherer ancestors ate a wide range of raw plants, plus a great variety of animal food which included shellfish, birds, rodents, and molluscs.

The introduction of cereal crops, milk, sugar, tea, and coffee, and the pollution of foods by agrochemicals and food additives, are all very recent changes in our diet. Our metabolism and digestion have adapted to these changes with time, but logically the foods that are most likely to give trouble if one's adaptation breaks down are those recently introduced. Wild animals, unlike intensively-reared ones, have little saturated fats, and no chemical residues. And because the hunter-gatherer ate a wide variety of things according to the seasons, he or she did not eat the same few things every day throughout the year.

So the modern version of the Stone Age Diet aims to cut out the foods *most likely* to cause trouble.

Stone Age Diet

Allowed	Not Allowed
All meats and fish (fresh or frozen)	Grains (wheat, oats, rye, corn, rice, barley)
Fruit	Sugar – all kinds
Vegetables (fresh)	Milk and milk products
Potatoes	Butter and margarine
Fresh shelled nuts	Tea, coffee, alcohol
Pulses	Anything tinned, smoked or processed
Spring water (glass-bottled)	Eggs
Pure vegetable oil	Dried fruit
Salt	Tap water
Milk-free margarine	

This system works well if you are not allergic to any of the foods on the 'allowed' list. It is quite possible to follow the Stone Age Diet for months and have complete nutrition. The main things to test, if two weeks or longer on the Stone Age Diet have improved your symptoms, are eggs, milk and its products, tap water, and some grains. A good grain to test early is rice, as it is less likely to cause symptoms than wheat or rye. Eggs are important to test early, as they are an excellent food; and rice, if safe, provides another carbohydrate. Sugar, tea, coffee, alcohol and processed foods are unimportant nutritionally.

If tap water causes a reaction, after testing on its own, then consider getting a water filter which removes the chlorine, lead, aluminium and nitrates. There are cheap ones which need a filter cartridge changed every month, and expensive ones which are plumbed into the main tap. Bottled spring water can be used on outings, but is expensive to use all the time. People living in rural areas with clean air can collect rain-water, but this still needs to be filtered.

Of the grains, wheat (in the UK) and corn (in the USA) are most likely to cause problems. You may be sensitive to the gluten, which is protein, or intolerant of the husk or bran. Some people with wheat intolerance can manage one slice of unprocessed white bread a day or twice a week, but get symptoms if they go back to four slices of wholemeal bread a day. Oats have less gluten, and if tolerated are a better source of fibre than wheat. Rice is rarely allergenic, perhaps because it is not part of our staple diet, and is low in gluten. Unrefined rice is a good substitute for wheat as a starch. There are less common, gluten-free grains – e.g. tapioca, buckwheat – that can also be substituted for wheat.

Cytotoxic Testing

A sample of blood is taken, and the white blood cells are separated out. The white cells are exposed to a range of foods and chemicals, and their reaction is examined under a microscope. The reactions are graded: No reaction; a mild reaction (the cells change shape); severe reaction (the cells die). The correlation between the results of the test and improvement following avoidance is fairly good, but the test is expensive and can only be performed at a few specialized centres. It tends to give a long list of allergens; however in practice one avoids the items which have given a severe or moderate reaction. One advantage is that chemicals can be tested for, whereas an elimination diet only sorts out foods.

Intradermal Testing and Neutralization Technique

This procedure is used by several clinical ecologists. It is expensive and time-consuming, and patients can have reactions which last for hours and confuse subsequent tests.

A minute dose of a solution of test substance in saline is injected into the skin, to raise a small bleb. The diameter of the bleb is measured, and after exactly two minutes the bleb is examined again. If it has increased in size, particularly if there is redness of the surrounding skin, or symptoms in the patient, this indicates a positive reaction. Successive diluted doses of the test substances are injected and measured, until a dilution is reached which causes no reaction. This commonly 'switches off' any symptoms, and calms the reaction in previous blebs. This is then recorded as the *neutralizing dilution*, or end point.

The patient is given drops or injections made up of the neutralizing strengths of the major antigens to use daily. This can be useful for a multiple-allergic subject, who can eat a wider range of foods with this protection. It is also valuable for severely chemically-allergic people, who react to minute amounts of chemicals that cannot be avoided in their environment.

The disadvantages are: a) the time needed to test for everything (one may spend a whole morning reaching the end point of one test substance!), and b) the end points may change after a few weeks, and the desensitizing drops may have to be worked out over and over again.

The mechanism by which this neutralization and desensitization works is probably electrical, as in highly diluted amounts there may be no original molecules left, as in homoeopathic remedies.

Applied Kinesiology (the muscle weakness test)

In this test, which requires no sophisticated equipment, the test substance itself, or a vial containing a solution of it, is placed in contact with the patient, usually over the centre of the abdomen. The patient is lying relaxed, and first the strength of one or more arm muscles is assessed, then retested after the test substance has been placed in contact with the patient's skin. It is not a trial of strength, and very small movements are tested. If the patient reacts to the item being tested, there is an immediate perceptible weakness in his or her muscles.

This method is fairly accurate in a skilled tester, but not everyone can develop this skill. It has the advantage of being non-invasive, quick, and does not produce unpleasant symptoms. With a skilled practitioner, the test has almost 100 per cent reproducability if a patient is tested on consecutive days. The patient should not know what substance is being tested each time.

Treating Food and Chemical Allergies

1. Avoid allergens where possible
2. Correct any nutrient deficiencies, and take supplements to strengthen the immune system
3. Desensitize by using neutralizing drops or injections
4. Enzyme Potentiated Desensitization (EPD)
5. Oral sodium cromoglycate – Nalcrom

Avoidance

For the majority of allergic people, avoidance of a few main foods, and cleaning up the chemical environment as far as possible, combined with nutritional measures, is best. If a major food allergen, such as wheat, is avoided for six months or so, the patient may become less sensitive and may be able to tolerate it if eaten in small amounts once or twice a week. If it is eaten daily and in increasing amounts, then a masked allergy may develop again.

Some allergies are fixed for life, and a long spell of avoidance does not change the sensitivity. There is often some enzyme deficiency associated with these allergies. Most patients find out if they have a life-long allergy to something eaten rarely such as strawberries or shellfish.

Milk allergy is commonly caused by a deficiency of lactase, the enzyme needed to digest lactose. This is usually life-long, is very common in Asians and Africans, and occurs in about 30 per cent of Europeans. Lactose intolerance sometimes develops following some gastro-intestinal infection, such as a bug called Giardia Lamblia (commonly picked up overseas), and also entero-viruses.

Some milk-sensitive people can tolerate milk if it has been treated with a lactose-reducing enzyme. Other milk sensitivities may be reactions to cow's milk protein, in which case the patient may be able to tolerate goat's or sheep's milk. If you are allergic to cow's milk, it is worth asking for separate tests for milk protein and lactose in allergy tests.

Often, avoidance of one or two foods will reduce the overall load and allow you to eat other things to which you are less sensitive. If the less sensitive foods are eaten no more than once every four days, or perhaps twice a week, there is less chance of a masked allergy developing. This is the principle of the Rotation Diet, which can be used both for managing and diagnosing allergies.

The Rotation Diet means you have different foods each day and allow four days before eating something again. Because of cross-sensitivity, a strict Rotation Diet includes members of the same food family in the four-day rule – e.g. if you eat chicken, neither it nor eggs must be eaten for the next four days. A Rotation Diet can be interesting to create on paper, using columns for food groups for each day. In practice it can be quite tedious, and you cannot use up leftovers the next day. It can be quite unworkable if you have to cater for the rest of the family, and makes eating out very awkward (as do most exclusion diets).

Enzyme Potentiated Desensitization (EPD)

This technique was developed by Dr Len McEwan, lately at St Mary's Hospital, London.

A mixture of minute doses of highly purified antigens is combined with an enzyme called *Beta-glucuronidase*, which potentiates the effects of the antigens, plus two other chemicals. This solution is introduced in one of two ways: It can be injected into the skin, to raise a small bleb, or it can be placed in contact with the skin on the patient's inner forearm in a small cup, the skin having been scratched beforehand to break the superficial layers. The solution of antigens and enzyme is left in contact with the skin for 24 hours, or less if a severe reaction develops.

A great number of antigens can be included in the mixture, maybe 70 or more, so it is not necessary to have established the patient's individual sensitivities.

EPD is repeated at monthly intervals for three to four months, but the benefits (increasing tolerance to foods) do not develop for six to twelve months after starting treatment. When it does work, the improvement seems to be permanent, unlike desensitizing drops or injections. EPD is expensive, however, and the results are not instant; nor is it available at many centres, few of these in the NHS. However, those who complete the course report good results which are more permanent than is true of other methods of desensitization.

EPD has now been tested in double-blind trials for hay fever, ulcerative colitis and childhood hyperactivity. The EPD trial for hay fever gave a dramatic improvement in patients after only one EPD injection.

Sodium Cromoglycate (Nalcrom)

This drug is better known by asthmatics, who inhale it from a puffer to prevent allergic asthma attacks. The drug works by blocking the reaction of certain cells (called *mast* cells) to the antigen, so that the chemical substances (including histamine) which cause the allergic effects – inflammation, wheezing, headaches, etc. – are not released. Mast cells exist scattered in the membranes lining the nose, throat, lung airways, and also the gut.

Nalcrom can be taken in capsules just before meals, and seems to be effective in preventing food allergy reactions in about two-thirds of the patients who try it. It is not a substitute for sensible avoidance of main food offenders, but could be very useful to someone who is allergic to many foods; also if the allergic person copes well at home, but has problems travelling or visiting others. It is only available on prescription, comes in 100 mg capsules, and the dosage for an adult is 100–200 mg three times daily. It is safe, although occasionally causes side-effects such as nausea, joint pains or rashes.

Suggested Supplements for Allergic People

First, ensure that any supplements you obtain are free from gluten, sugar, yeast, grains, and colourings.

The regime suggested for M.E. (page 168) is quite suitable.

The main deficiencies that occur in very allergic people are of B vitamins, pantothenic acid, iron, zinc, magnesium and essential fatty acids.

Dealing with bowel bug overgrowths such as Candida (see Chapter 13) may improve food intolerances quite dramatically.

A Word of Caution

If you have lost weight with M.E., are already underweight, or have severe symptoms, do *not* undertake elimination diets without specialized medical supervision. By further reducing your nutritional intake, you may become worse. If possible, seek advice from a medically-trained clinical ecologist, or a hospital specialist.

If you want to try and sort things for yourself and haven't got medical help, a suggested routine is:

First – follow the diet guidelines outlined in Chapter 11, avoid all chemicals in food, and take the suggested nutritional supplements. This may improve your symptoms after two months.

Second – if you suspect food allergies, try either the Stone Age Diet, eating plenty of vegetables, meat, fish and fruit, or cut out completely either wheat, or cow's milk, one at a time, as these are the most common offenders.

Third – reduce other possible allergens as much as possible, i.e. any chemicals around you.

Chapter 15

Chemical Sensitivity

This problem seems to be increasing. You only have to consider the vast array of products made from petro-chemicals (hydrocarbons) which have become part of twentieth-century living, to see that we cannot possibly expect humans to have adapted to them in such a short time.

Rachel Carson's classic book *Silent Spring*, written back in 1962, was a chilling forecast of the price we may have to pay for tampering with the environment. Talking about the effect of DDT and other pesticides on living creatures and food chains, she said, 'It looks as if we will go on swallowing these chemicals whether we like it or not and their real effect may not be seen for another twenty or thirty years.'

Most M.E. people seem to have an increased degree of sensitivity to chemicals compared to when they were well, and chemical allergy goes with food allergy. Some reactions are obvious: for example, someone who gets a headache and watering eyes when they open the morning newspaper is probably sensitive to printer's ink. However, there may be more insidious symptoms, harder to relate to their cause. Someone who is very sensitive may be unwell on days when the wind blows from the direction of some chemical factory 30 miles away. The presence of a smoker in the household may cause chronic worsening of symptoms in a susceptible non-smoker. A minute gas leak from an old cooker can make you ill.

Other than moving to a remote place by the sea, drinking spring water and growing your own food organically, you may feel that you have little control over your environment. You can, however, support pressure groups such as Friends of the Earth, Greenpeace, or write to your Member of Parliament about environmental issues. Nearer to home, there is a lot you can do to clean up your immediate environment.

Chemicals that Cause Problems

Hydrocarbons, or Fossil Fuels

Petrol, diesel, oils – (from cars and trucks, boat engines)
  Paraffin (kerosene) – as used in kerosene stoves
  Natural or calor gas – (from central heating, gas cookers)
  Coal, coke, anthracite – (coal-fired stoves, open fires)
  Wood, charcoal – (wood smoke, barbecues, stoves)

Hydrocarbon Derivatives

People who are sensitive to the things listed above are usually also affected by hydrocarbon products:
  Plastics – wrappings, bottles, clingfilm, plastic food boxes, plastic furnishings
  Synthetic textiles – nylon, terylene, dralon, polyester, in clothing, carpets and upholstery
  Paints, varnish, solvents – as found in newly-decorated buildings
  Aerosol propellants – these are numerous and widespread, being found in hair spray, deodorants, insect sprays, air 'fresheners', etc.
  Detergents, polishes, and cleaning fluids
  Cosmetics, perfumes, scented soaps, and wax candles

Phenol Products

Carbolic acid – this is pure phenol
  Dettol and other antiseptics
  Many preservatives
  Pesticides, herbicides

Polyurethane foam
Dyes
Bakelite and hard plastics

Formaldehyde

Found in dyes, fabric finishes, and proofings in textiles (if you feel unwell in a large clothing store, it is formaldehyde affecting you)

Traffic fumes
Fertilizers, insecticides, foam rubber
Fabric conditioner
Paper manufacture, printing ink, photography
Most building materials, cavity wall insulation
Many other products

Gardening and Agricultural Chemicals

These are too numerous to list. Many are now banned, but can still be found lurking in garden sheds. They include herbicides, which kill unwanted plants, although they usually break down quickly.

Fertilizers may be safe for plants if diluted, but may be toxic to us while undiluted.

Pesticides are potentially the most harmful. DDT, although banned, builds up in food chains and has been detected even in the Arctic ice, it is now so widespread. Organophosphates kill insects by interfering with their nerve function. They are probably the lethal component in chemical bombs, such as those used in the massacre of a Kurdish community in northern Iraq. Some humans are very susceptible to even traces of organophosphates, and sheep farmers in particular are at risk as a result of skin contact with sheep dip. Symptoms of organophosphate poisoning can linger for years, and may resemble M.E. – headaches, muscular weakness and exhaustion, nausea, sweating, loss of co-ordination, loss of cognitive brain function, etc. The main sources of exposure, if you are not a sheep dipper, are household insect sprays or being near crop fields that have just been sprayed.

Food Colourings

The following foods usually have synthetic colourings:

    Glacé cherries, coloured ice creams, sweets, lollipops
    Orangeade, lemonade, fruit-flavoured drinks
    Yellow cheeses, coloured cakes and icing
    Canned soft drinks
    Many processed foods

The correct procedure is to check the label when buying foods. The items listed above should be avoided by people with M.E. anyway.

Colourings in Medicines

This source of potential trouble is easy to overlook. Many medicines are still coloured or flavoured with synthetic chemicals, some of which are banned in countries other than the UK. If a medicine you really need is suspiciously coloured, your pharmacist should be able to enquire of the manufacturers what the contents are.

Chemicals in Tobacco Smoke

You need not be a smoker to be affected by the fumes from other people's cigarettes, pipes or cigars. This smoke contains many chemicals, and a sensitive person can even be affected by traces lingering on clothes. If you or someone near you smokes, then avoiding all the other sources of chemical pollution may be a waste of time. You are entitled to a smoke-free place at work, and *you must make your home a smoke-free zone if you are serious about improving your health*.

Minimizing Chemical Pollution

On Your Person

Wear natural fibres if possible. Avoid fabrics with special finishes, and clothes that have to be dry-cleaned – or at least air them well after they've been dry-cleaned. Make sure the washing is well rinsed, use soap powders or flakes or ecologically safe detergents; avoid fabric softeners. When buying clothes, look for cottons, pure wools, or silk, and if a garment has any odour don't buy it, or wash it several times before wearing it. Cotton/terylene mixes are better than pure nylon.

Do not use perfume, aftershaves, deodorants, scented soaps or talcum power, or synthetic bath bubbles. Avoid hair sprays and scented shampoos.

Women wearing make-up should use natural products, such as The Body Shop range and similar. Transforming a M.E.-ravaged face can be morale-boosting!

In Your Home
You and others around you must not smoke.

In the bathroom, remove air fresheners, toilet deodorizers, and all cleaning agents. The bath and WC can be cleaned with the least smelly agents possible, and these can be kept in a cupboard somewhere else, or outside. It is a myth, fostered by advertising agencies, that artificial smells of 'pine' or 'meadow freshness' equal hygiene. Women brought up during a less chemically-inclined era will remember that bathrooms could be kept clean without all these smells.

Look under the kitchen sink, and see what cleaning agents you can jettison. Those you decide to keep, such as ecologic washing-up liquid and sink cleaner, keep tightly sealed. Spray furniture polish, instant floor cleaners, insect killer or fresh air sprays should all go out. In summer, old-fashioned sticky fly-paper can be quite efficient at keeping down flies. There is little that cannot be cleaned with water, soap, or bicarbonate of soda, and the best air freshener is an open window. It is better to have a grubby home than a shiny, scented house with ill occupants.

Paints and solvents should be stored outside, in the shed or garage. Plans for redecorating should be postponed until you are either better or can go away while it is being done and not return until the smell has cleared.

It is probably not practical to rip up all wall-to-wall foam-backed carpets, but if you are chemically allergic it might be worth taking up such a carpet from your bedroom and keeping just the old linoleum that may be underneath, or having bare floorboards with woollen rugs or carpets that can be shaken outside. Another benefit of bare floors is a reduction of house dust; fitted carpets can never be properly cleaned, and they also harbour house dust mites, a cause of asthma.

Very sensitive ill people find benefit from creating one room in the house which is as chemical-free as possible – a 'safe haven', with natural cotton curtains, no plastics, no treated furniture, no foam, and no treated wallpaper. Many modern wallpapers are treated with fungicides, and cause trouble for some time.

If you are replacing furniture, try and avoid foam-filled furnishings with synthetic or imitation leather covers. Basically, anything new or that smells is likely to be chemically treated. The best furnishings are of wood or metal, with cotton or wool covers, and kapok (a cotton-like material) cushions.

One problem area is the bed. Should you have feather- or foam filled pillows? Good-quality feather pillows are better, provided you are not allergic to feathers. A lot of the allergic reactions to beds and bedding is due to the ubiquitous house dust mite, which establishes itself in all soft furnishings. Covering the mattress and pillows with finely woven cotton ticking helps. Washable wool or cotton blankets can be kept free of dust mites, and the best duvet would be feather-filled but also washable.

On the subject of house dust mites, vacuum cleaning can bring on symptoms. There are cleaners that can connect to an outside vent so that dust is not recycled into the room.

In the kitchen, avoid plastic food containers, bags or clingfilm. Greaseproof paper is better for wrapping.

Cooking utensils should be of stainless steel, pyrex, cast iron or enamelled ware. Aluminium pans are bad for anyone, as aluminium is poisonous and small amounts enter cooking food, especially stewed fruit. The non-stick linings of pans may seem convenient, but the chemicals they contain can contaminate your food. Also, when the non-stick surface deteriorates the food sticks and burns far worse than on an ordinary pan.

More difficult to get rid of in your home is a heating system that might be releasing minute quantities of fumes that are affecting you; nor may it be easy to find out whether the heating system is the true culprit. Most people in urban areas of the UK have North Sea gas heating – it is worth having your appliances thoroughly serviced regularly and tested for leaks. A gas cooker is relatively easy to replace with an electric one, as gas cookers are common sources of minute traces of gas, leaking from the pilot light.

One way to test if gas is causing a problem is to go and stay somewhere with no gas at all and see if you improve. On returning, if you can smell any trace of gas at all, you are probably sensitive to it. Most modern appliances give little trouble. Alternatively, you can switch off the gas at source for two weeks, ventilate the house well, and then see if any symptoms return when it is switched on again. This test may not be so clear as going away, as traces of gas persist from pipes and connections.

Many M.E. sufferers seem to get worse in winter. I wonder if being indoors most of the day with central heating and lack of ventilation is as much to blame as is lack of sunshine and daylight? Indoor pollution is worse than outdoor pollution, unless when you step out the door you are faced by a busy road, or a chemical factory. At least outdoor pollution gets blown away sometimes by a good wind. A lot of people never open any windows in the house, for fear of burglars or losing heat. But even in winter, each room should be ventilated once a day for a while, especially on windy days, when the outside air is cleaner.

Other sources of indoor pollution are wood preservatives, certain cavity wall insulations (foam), tobacco smoke, damp and mould (adequate ventilation should prevent these), portable gas heaters, coal- or oil-fired stoves, and insecticides, as well as air-conditioning units and integrally-built garages.

Televisions and VDU screens, when in operation, give off formaldehyde from their plastic components. They may also produce electromagnetic and other radiations, which are harmful to M.E. sufferers, and indeed to everyone. This may be why so many M.E. people cannot tolerate exposure to much television. One person commented that he had the same ill effects by sitting in front of a TV with his eyes blindfolded as he had if he watched the programme. His symptoms were head-aches, increased mental 'fog' and blurred vision for up to 24 hours after exposure to TV for any length of time.

A solution for users of computers, whether at work or at home, is to attach a special screen which blocks off the harmful rays. An ionizer in the room also seems to help.

A fairly drastic step is to move house, if there seems to be something harmful in your home or neighbour-hood that cannot be corrected. Obviously there is no point in giving up a home with gas heating only to move to a quiet country cottage surrounded by crop fields which are regularly sprayed! So, if such a step is taken, it is important to look for somewhere with electric heating, or a boiler well away from the house, in a relatively unpolluted area away from busy roads.

With smoke-free enforcement in most cities, urban air may be cleaner than in some parts of the countryside, as mentioned above, if you can find a quiet area with plenty of greenery. Old houses may be unsafe because of treatment for timber and dry rot. Probably the best homes ecologically (in the UK) are those built between 1920 and 1960.

Combating an Acute Reaction

Drink a glass of water containing one gm of vitamin C and one level teaspoon of bicarbonate of soda. Repeat the vitamin C if necessary, at hourly intervals, and continue to drink lots of fluids for 24 hours. This helps to neutralize the reaction, and gives a boost to the white cells and adrenals. Whatever the mechanism, this remedy does help, so keep vitamin C handy at home and if travelling. This mixture is useful to take on aeroplanes – air travel involves chemical exposure both on planes and in modern airport terminals.

At home, change your clothes and have a shower, to remove traces of the chemical from your clothes and skin. Go outside (if inside), or open a window and breathe deeply of clean air. If in a car, shut all windows and vents, and try and get away from whatever it is – crop sprays, road works, or a queue of buses. Bach Rescue Remedy drops (see page 236) are invaluable, and can be taken for any sort of collapse or shock, whether chemical, emotional or sheer physical exhaustion. Together with glucose sweets, and some vitamin C and bicarb, a small bottle of Rescue Remedy should be part of every M.E. sufferer's first-aid kit. I have found all these things essential on occasions when travelling, when one's expectations of endurance tend to far exceed reality.

Desensitization

Some clinical ecologists treat very chemically-sensitive patients in a special ecologically safe unit, where everything is done to create a chemical-free environment. Patients often improve dramatically while in these surroundings, and can return home with a supply of desensitizing drops or injections.

This is fine, so long as the patient also takes steps to clean up his or her home as much as possible, to deal with any likely Candida infection, and to correct any nutritional deficiencies. But chemical sensitivity will return after a time, unless the underlying immune dysfunction improves.

Avoidance of all possible allergens will help the immune system, and so should be attempted by M.E. sufferers as part of their self-help plan.

The following history is of someone who found chemical avoidance helpful. It also illustrates that many health workers still do not understand the symptoms of M.E.

Mrs I . C., aged 28, Ex-hairdresser.

Her illness started in 1982, suddenly. She has been ill since then.

'I believe long-term exposure to chemicals at work – hairsprays, perms, bleaches etc. – whittled away at my immune system over the years; then in the year previous to the onset I was working long hours. So when I went down with the infection it was severe, and I think my powers of recovery were not a quarter of what they should have been.

'My symptoms were, and are: feeling very ill, muscle weakness and pain, strange sensations in my head, pain in all my muscles, especially in my thighs, excessive perspiration, giddiness, cold feet and hands, wheezing, palpitations, pain as though I had ''acid'' coursing through my veins.'

Mrs C. had a muscle biopsy and blood tests done two years after the onset; the muscle biopsy was abnormal, and the diagnosis was myalgic encephalomyelitis. She also had myocarditis three years ago. She has been virtually bedridden and permanently fatigued for most of the last five years. During the last year there has been some improvement, however:

'Ridding my home of all chemicals has produced a dramatic improvement. After being totally collapsed and bedridden for over a year an M.E. sufferer, also a patient of Dr Jean Monro, told me to move house and clear out at least my bedroom of all allergens or I would be bedridden for the rest of my life. It made sense. My ex-home had been totally renovated and sprayed with fungicide (for dry rot) and pesticide (for woodworm). Also I lived in a top-floor flat on a busy road, my carpets were foam-backed, the furniture was chipboard and hardboard. I surrounded myself with perfumes and spent a fortune on bath oils and foams. We were advised to buy a home which was 15-to-20 years old (any older and it would most likely have been sprayed and damp-treated).

'We lifted the carpet in the bedroom of our new home, and luckily there were cream-coloured, hard vinyl tiles underneath which cleaned up well. We use all 100 per cent cotton sheets and night attire, and got rid of our modern furniture. I gave away all my perfume, and now buy *Simple* toiletries. I'm phasing out my clothes, which are made of synthetic fabrics. I don't allow anyone to smoke in my house, and I ask friends and family not to wear perfume, aftershave, or hairspray when visiting.

'A friend was wearing hairspray when visiting recently. I didn't like to say anything at first, but after 1½ hours I went from being able to sit quite easily to collapsing and unable to hold myself up – I could hardly believe the effect it had on me! After she'd gone it took two hours for the air to clear with the door open – when it did clear and I had gulped in lots of fresh air I could sit once again.

'I would advise all bedridden or severely affected people to take the same advice, remembering all family members must switch to unscented toiletries.

'In June of this year I had a dreadful experience. I was horrifically unwell and living with my parents, as we had just sold our flat. My husband had just started his new job and was in agony with three slipped discs in his back. I was totally incapacitated and unable to wash myself or get to the toilet unaided. In desperation I wrote to Dr W. at –– Hospital, and they took me in. I was carried out on a stretcher, as I couldn't sit or stand. The first day wasn't too bad, except the nurses wanted me to walk a very long corridor to the toilet – it was agony, I couldn't hold myself up.

'I tried to explain that I couldn't sit up in bed for my meals, yet they wanted me to sit at a table. The staff could see how disabled I was because they had trundled me away in an ambulift for a bath, in which I just slumped, totally unable to move. On the third day they wanted me to go to the gym for physiotherapy. I tried again to explain how terribly ill I felt, and that I couldn't even sit up. I felt sucked to the bed like an iron filing to a magnet.

'It was the last straw when the nurse said to me at lunchtime "Do you *want* to sit at the table?" I just lost control, and screamed at her in floods of tears, and told every one of them that I was not trying to be uncooperative, that I was not a lazy creature who enjoyed lying in bed. The doctor called me selfish, and said I had an abnormal attitude and that the reason I had been bedridden for over a year was because I had put down "clamps" and was afraid of trying. I realized just how much this research hospital knew about M.E.: Nothing.

'I just want to forget it all now and concentrate on getting better, which I feel quietly confident about. I believe our healing to a large extent comes from within ourselves, and that self-help should mean exactly that. I have kept a diary since I've been ill, and have come to a number of conclusions about this illness which I am trying to get down on paper, hoping to help others.

'Things which have helped me include relaxation tapes, home-help (I had over 25 phone calls in response to advert!), my personal stereo (ideal for listening to relaxation tapes, etc. when bedridden), massage – various books available – and meditation, hot baths (but not *too* hot) – helps inflammation and vein pain, fresh air – as much as possible, Christian counselling – ask at your local Christian bookshop for this service (good for Christians and non-Christians alike), and Christian healing – local church prayer groups usually have a healing ministry. Also the book *Chemical Children*, which is about chemical avoidance.'

Suggested Further Reading
Rachel Carson, *Silent Spring*, (Penguin, 1962, Pelican, 1983).

Chapter 16

Treatments and Hazards

Drugs

M.E. patients need to be very cautious about taking medicines for various reasons: so many sufferers become hypersensitive to drugs, and in some there may be a problem, if the liver is at all affected, in breaking down and disposing of a drug. Also drugs affecting the nervous system may produce quite bizarre effects, sometimes the opposite of what is intended.

A good rule is to discuss with your doctor any medicine you may be prescribed. You need to know exactly what it is – its name and purpose, the symptoms it is supposed to treat, how to take it, and for how long. Report any possible side-effects as soon as possible. Various self-medications that can be bought at a chemist's, and which for you were once harmless, may now cause side-effects or allergic reactions if you have M.E. Beware of medicines or pills that have colourings which cause a reaction, and be aware that many cough medicines also contain sugar or alcohol.

Drugs to be Avoided (Unless Essential)

Tranquillizers
Tranquillizers include drugs such as Valium, Librium, and Ativan. These can be addictive, can make depression worse, and do not do anything to correct underlying brain disturbance.

Antibiotics
Broad-spectrum antibiotics in particular should be

avoided. Ideally, proof of a bacterial infection should be obtained first, such as by a urine culture or throat swab (for suspected urine or throat infections); if an antibiotic is needed, hopefully your doctor will prescribe one specifically for that infection, for a limited length of time. The sensible M.E. patient who develops an infection will take measures to help his or her body's natural resistance, such as taking extra vitamin C, zinc, and vitamin A, and getting extra rest and plenty of fluids.

If you require a course of antibiotics, take the complete course; a half-hearted course leads to more trouble as the germs may come back, and may develop resistance to that antibiotic. Restore the friendly bugs in your gut, which will have been depleted by the antibiotic, by taking probiotics for at least two weeks after the antibiotics are finished.

Steroids

If you are already taking cortico-steroids, i.e. cortisone, prednisolone or similar, *do not stop taking them*, but consult your GP or specialist about the need for them. Steroids may cause temporary improvement of symptoms in many conditions, including asthma, multiple sclerosis, arthritis, ulcerative colitis and fibromyalgia.

However, this dramatic improvement happens because the body's own supply of cortisone is boosted artificially; this can dampen down the symptoms which result from allergic reactions (e.g. asthma), or from auto-immune diseases. Short-term benefits are outweighed by the longer-term effects of steroids: laziness of the adrenal-cortex glands in making one's own cortisone, which leads to poor response to stress and infection, and to increasing dependence on the steroid drug as the source of cortisone. Suppression of symptoms does nothing to correct the underlying problem which produced them, a problem with many drugs. It may also mask other serious conditions, such as TB or cancer. Natural cortisone levels fluctuate during 24 hours, and this natural response to the body's needs cannot be duplicated by regular pills. Other side-effects can be high blood-pressure, fluid retention, loss of calcium from bones – leading to osteoporosis – muscle weakness, stomach ulcers, and mental symptoms of depression or euphoria. Also any Candida yeast infections flare up.

A person who has been on steroids for more than a few weeks must not suddenly stop them. If long-term treatment is to be stopped, the dose has to be lowered very gradually over a period of time, and under medical supervision.

There *are* conditions where steroids save lives, and for some people life-long replacement steroid therapy is essential. However, steroids are *not* recommended for people with M.E., as the side-effects strongly outweigh any short-term suppression of symptoms.

Oral Contraceptives
'The pill' was hailed as the ideal contraceptive. However, certain long-term problems from its use have become recognized. Female hormones are related to cortisone in their chemical structure, and artificial levels can have some of the effects of steroids – weight gain, mental changes, and Candida yeast overgrowth.

Oral contraceptives also lead to depletion of zinc, and raised copper levels. There is increased tendency to allergies, migraines, blood clotting, high blood-pressure, and depression. Some of the mental symptoms may be due to the disturbance of B-vitamin metabolism by the pill, and to the change in the zinc/copper ratio. So women with M.E., who may have enough problems with depression, thrush, and blood-sugar, should not create further problems by taking the pill.

There is evidence to show that the long-term effects of being on the pill for several years include a greater risk of allergies and less resistance to infections, indicating some changes in immune response.

Anaesthetics and Surgery

All anaesthetic agents are drugs with powerful effects on the central nervous system. Any after-effects may be more severe for an M.E. sufferer. I know of two cases where the effect of a muscle paralysing drug (routinely used in anaesthesia after you have gone to sleep, to allow a tube to be safely passed down the airway) has taken an abnormally long time to wear off after the operation. Since in M.E. there appears to be some disturbance of the neuro-transmitters between nerve cells, and also some disturbance of muscle function, it is not surprising that a routine anaesthetic may cause problems. Obviously there are occasions when surgery is essential; you would not wish to delay operating on acute appendicitis or a broken leg.

If surgery is really needed, it is important that you tell the anaesthetist you have M.E., and describe any problems you may have with muscles, walking, co-ordination, and brain symptoms. Then he or she can make adjustments and use the most appropriate drugs, in lower doses if necessary.

Of course, any operation is stressful and may bring on some kind of relapse. If it is unavoidable, then try to make provision for extra care and rest in the convalescent period, and take extra vitamin C, zinc, vitamin A and all B vitamins for a few weeks after surgery. Allow yourself plenty of time to recover. Non-essential surgical procedures should be postponed until the M.E. is better, or is stable, which may be well before your turn comes upon the waiting list! Remember that hundreds of people with M.E. do have operations safely each year.

Local Anaesthetic

Many M.E. sufferers report increased sensitivity to local anaesthetic. It may be a reaction to the adrenaline which is often combined with the anaesthetic, and it is wise to ask the surgeon to use a local that does not contain added adrenaline. Several instances have been recorded of M.E. people collapsing or losing consciousness after local anaesthesia for dental procedures. On the other hand, many muscle biopsies have been performed on M.E. patients, with no ill effect from the local anaesthetic. So the reactions experienced in the dentist's chair may be partly due to stress caused by 'dentist phobia', or to the dose used, or to the site of injection being closer to the brain.

Whatever the reasons, non-urgent dental treatment, apart from scaling and cleaning, is probably not a good idea while you are unwell with M.E. Candida often lurks in the mouth and in gum crevices, so good preventative mouth and gum hygiene is extremely important. You may find that your gums' health improves after improving your diet and increasing your vitamin C intake. But tooth abscess or any chronic mouth sepsis must be treated, with penicillin and dental surgery if needed, as any septic focus in the body damages health and will worsen M.E.

Mercury Toxicity – Is it Relevant?
Talking of dental treatment, another reason why some M.E. patients report a relapse following dental work involving fillings may be to do with mercury sensitivity. This is a very controversial topic. Although the use of mercury amalgam is being abandoned in some European countries, there is a reluctance in the British dental profession to look closely at mercury's hazards.

What Are the Facts?
We know that mercury is extremely poisonous. It is used in a mixture with silver, tin, copper and zinc, containing about 50 per cent mercury. Once the amalgam has been installed in a tooth, there is no proof that some of the mercury does not escape in the form of vapour and enter the body. When the fillings are ground, as is done when chewing, some mercury does escape as vapour, and this can enter the saliva and be swallowed, and can be

converted into methyl mercury by the action of bacteria in the mouth and in the gut. Methyl mercury is much more toxic than elemental mercury.

Because there is more than one metal in the mouth and there is liquid in the form of saliva, a small but measurable electric current is continuously generated in the mouth. This is something that gradually corrodes the amalgam, together with foodstuffs and chemicals and physical wearing away by chewing. All amalgam fillings gradually deteriorate, some have to be replaced after five to ten years. So where has the mercury gone?

The electric potentials between teeth and their surrounding saliva can be measured using a *milli-ammeter*. Some of the symptoms possibly due to the electric current in the mouth, which has been measured as 900 mv or more, include a metallic taste in the mouth, increased salivation, irritability, pins and needles or pain in the face, and severe depression. The roots of teeth, particularly in the upper jaw, pass close to main nerves, and the impulses passing along nerves can be affected by local electric currents.

Research has demonstrated that mercury can affect central nervous system functioning, and also has a bad effect on the immune system. It was demonstrated in 1984 that removal of amalgam fillings resulted in a rise in circulating T lymphocytes, whose numbers fell when the amalgam was reinserted. This may be due to hypersensitivity to amalgam fillings. There is certainly plenty of documented evidence of the undesirable results of having such a toxic metal in the mouth. I am not suggesting that mercury toxicity is a *cause* of M.E. or CFS, but it may contribute to damage to the immune system and increase susceptibility to developing immune dysfunction diseases. For those who would like to pursue this matter further, I recommend the book *The Toxic Time Bomb*, by Sam Ziff.

The problem for someone who has been diagnosed as having M.E. or CFS, who is getting worse and has a lot of old amalgam fillings, is this: Do you ask your dentist to take them all out, and replace them with one of the newer metal-free fillings?

There are several snags about this:

1. The replacement is not available on the NHS, and will therefore be costly.
2. You need to have evidence first that the amalgam is causing trouble, which is hard to find. However, it is possible to have tests done which show if the mercury is leaking out, and if you are allergic to it. These tests are only available from a few dentists, however.
3. The process of removing amalgam causes a great release of mercury, and usually the patient feels much worse for some days, maybe longer. In other words, it may induce a severe relapse.
4. The removal needs to be done by a dentist who is aware of the hazards, with special precautions taken to minimize swallowing and inhaling the amalgam. The fillings need to be removed in a particular sequence, depending on which ones are causing the greatest reaction.
5. Some of the replacement materials may cause problems. Ideally the patient needs to be tested for sensitivity to different substitute materials beforehand.
6. Because it is a procedure which causes worsening of symptoms, it is essential to take extra immune-boosting supplements (vitamins A and C, zinc, and calcium pantothenate) before and for several weeks afterwards.

There is an urgent need for more research into the connections between mercury amalgam fillings and immune functioning, the nervous system, and indeed the whole physiology of the body. There are no figures to show if the percentage of people with amalgam fillings is significantly different between M.E. patients and healthy controls.

In the meantime, the advice to M.E. patients about changing dental fillings is this: *Do not rush into having your amalgam fillings removed*, especially if you are really ill. If you start to get better, and feel you would like advice about it, contact the Dental Society for Clinical Nutrition (see Appendix A).

Immunizations

An immunization is a procedure in which the body's immune system is stimulated to produce an antibody to a specific infection; so that if the virus or bacteria causing the infection enters the body at a later date, the white blood cells will recognize it and produce lots more antibodies very quickly. The antigen which stimulates antibody production is usually a form of virus or bacteria which has been killed or changed to make it harmless. When smallpox immunization was given, a modified relative, called cowpox, was used.

The question of immunization for an M.E. sufferer arises in these circumstances:

- Before foreign travel – e.g. a typhoid, cholera, yellow-fever, or polio booster.
- To start or boost protection against tetanus, for going abroad, for gardeners and agricultural workers, or when there is a penetrating wound.
- Schoolchildren with M.E. who would normally be at the age to have BCG (for TB), rubella (only girls need this), or any booster vaccine.

Practically all M.E. people will have had childhood immunizations to protect against tetanus, diphtheria, polio, smallpox, BCG (for TB), and possibly measles, mumps and rubella.

If tetanus protection is advised because of a risky wound, this must be done, because tetanus is lethal. Tetanus toxoid is not derived from live germs, and therefore should be less likely to produce a reaction.

The main occasion when you may consider having an

immunization is before going abroad. Unless it is obligatory before entering the foreign country, the advice to M.E. patients is *don't have immunizations*.

Typhoid and cholera (commonly given together as TAB/cho) immunizations cause some reaction in all healthy people, and may lead to a severe reaction, a relapse, or possibly to no reaction at all, in someone with M.E. The lack of any reaction may mean that no immunity develops, yet the person, unaware of this, will eat and drink contaminated food in the belief that he or she is protected. It is better not to go to countries where there is a high risk of contracting enteric diseases; if you go, though, be scrupulously careful about hygiene: boil water before you drink or cook with it, and do not eat uncooked food in cafes. Anyway, typhoid and cholera injections do not protect against dysentery and hepatitis, which are just as easily picked up in many countries.

Immunizations are intended to stir up the immune system, but if the immune system is not functioning normally, one can end up with hypersensitive reactions, or incomplete immunity.

Some Useful Drugs

Ideally, it would be best to do without any drugs at all; however there are occasions when certain medicines can help tide one over a bad patch, and assist in dealing with troublesome symptoms. It is important to reduce pain, and also insomnia, as both of these are stresses that hinder recovery.

As you have probably found out, much of living with M.E. turns out to be based on compromise. I do not agree with purists who say that all conventional drugs are wrong; nor with narrow-minded doctors who prescribe drugs with possible side-effects, but condemn all 'alternative treatments' (usually through ignorance) which in general are safer and gentler than drugs. The rigidly obsessive M.E. patient whose life is dominated by strict rules is not going to be open to trying various therapies, nor to be aware of what suits him or her.

Sleeping Pills
If these are needed and other measures don't help, then one of the short-acting hypnotics is best, such as Temazepam or Triazolam, starting with a small dose. Some people worry about dependence on them, but to use them to achieve healing sleep is more sensible than nights of wakefulness followed by days of feeling exhausted. As you get better you can do without them. But sleeping pills may be less effective than tricyclics (see below).

Antihistamines
In small doses such as 2–4 mg twice daily, an antihistamine such as *Piriton* (chlorpheniramine) can be very helpful if there are many allergic symptoms, particularly the chronic explosive sneezing and streaming nose experienced by some sufferers. It causes a little sedation, but if taken at night, this is no disadvantage. Some newer antihistamines are non-sedative.

Nalcrom (Sodium Cromoglycate)
This may be helpful to prevent reactions in severely food-allergic patients, if they are in a situation where they cannot control their diet. One or two 100 mg capsules are taken before meals, either whole, or dissolved in water.

Painkillers
Avoid aspirin and compounds containing aspirin. Many people are sensitive to salycilates, and aspirin is now known to cause allergic responses and may be implicated in a hypersensitivity illness in children called Reye's syndrome. It is also irritating to the stomach. All the non-steroid anti-inflammatory drugs (e.g. ibuprofen) have the potential for stomach irritation, and should be taken with food.

Ibuprofen (Brufen) is an anti-inflammatory that can be used for headaches, joint pain and period pain.

Paracetamol has fewer side-effects than aspirin. Again a small dose should be tried, such as ½ or 1 tablet, instead of 2 tablets.

A good remedy for pain is vitamin C, 500 mg every hour. It has anti-prostaglandin effects similar to those of aspirin and anti-inflammatory drugs, and is much safer.

Antidepressants

Tricyclic antidepressants are closely related (chemically) to antihistamines. Although a controlled trial of tricyclics in treating M.E. is still awaited, the drug does seem to help some patients. The main benefit is improving the quality of sleep, probably by correcting the disturbance in non-REM sleep. A dose that is much less than that used to treat severe depression seems to help not only sleep, but also:

- Other brain functions – cognition, concentration, memory
- Muscle power (also reduces muscle spasms)
- Emotional lability (also reduces depressive symptoms)
- Some allergic reactions e.g. asthma, sneezing, as reported by some patients

As so many M.E. symptoms may result from disorder in neuro-transmitters (the chemical messengers between nerve cells), especially those that influence hypo-thalamic functions, it is not surprising that tricyclic drugs work in many patients. They work by increasing the level of certain brain peptides, such as serotonin.

I want to emphasize that these drugs do *not* suit *all* M.E. people, nor do they effect a cure for the majority who benefit from them.

Many M.E. patients do not tolerate tricyclics, often because the initial dose prescribed is too high (see also page 130). A tricyclic that has been tested on patients with 'fibromyalgia syndrome' (thought in the USA to be possibly identical to the myalgic form of CFS) is amitriptyline. When prescribed at only 10 or 20 mg nightly, it improves sleep and muscle pain and tenderness in fibromyalgia syndrome. There is more about tricyclic drugs in Chapter 10.

Tested Treatments

Essential Fatty Acids

In a trial in Glasgow (Behan, 1990), it was found that EFA supplements have beneficial effects on M.E. (see page 167).

The levels of essential fatty acids in the blood, which were abnormal at the start of the trial, returned to near normal after three months. EFAs have been shown to inhibit the production of cytokines and replication of viruses. The authors of the trial noted that no patients were cured, but that they could increase their activities and felt better.

Intravenous Immunoglobulin Therapy

In Australia (Lloyd et al., 1990), 49 patients with CFS were given either intravenous infusions of immunoglobulin (2 gm/kg/month) or a placebo for three months. After assessment, 43 per cent who had received immunoglobulin had improved, compared to 12 per cent of those given the placebo. At the start, 82 per cent of the patients were found to have abnormal cell-mediated hypersensitivity and/or reduced T-cells. In many of those who improved on Ig therapy, these abnormal immune test results returned to normal.

In another immunoglobulin trial, in the USA (Peterson et al., 1990), patients received either IgG (1 gm/kg) or a placebo every month for six months. In this trial there was no significant improvement in any patients, and side-effects occurred in a fifth of patients. The dose used was less than that in the Australian trial.

There seems to be a contradiction in the results of these two trials, and intravenous immunoglobulin is not yet recommended treatment, perhaps unless there is evidence of reduced levels of circulating IgG in the patient.

Magnesium injections
See page 164.

Treatments Used or Being Tested in the USA

Calcium Channel Blockers
These are already used to treat angina, high blood-pressure and migraine. When used to treat CFS they are thought to improve blood flow in the brain.

Ampligen
Ampligen is double-stranded RNA, which mimics the RNA in the immune system. It has both antiviral and immune-modifying effects, and may remove some block in the immune system which prevents it from recognizing virus.

A controlled trial of Ampligen, using 200 patients, was completed in July 1991. The results showed that Ampligen was an effective treatment for the severely debilitating form of chronic fatigue syndrome. Ampligen improved both the physical debility and the cognitive dysfunctions. There was no significant toxicity from Ampligen. Symptoms of low-grade fever and muscle and joint pain tended to improve with the treatment, and were probably due to the disease and not to Ampligen.

Unfortunately, in spite of this promising result, Ampligen is not yet a licensed drug in the USA. Hopefully further trials will convince the authorities there that this is a worthwhile treatment. Ampligen is not available for use outside clinical trials in the UK or other countries.

The Physician's Forum, issued by the CFIDS Association of USA (address in Appendix A), gives an overall account of all treatments in use or under trial for CFS in the USA.

Chapter 17

Homoeopathy and Other Therapies

If you suffer from an illness which goes on and on, for which conventional medicine has no answers, it is likely that you will look for help from the traditional forms of healing. The art of healing is as old as humanity, and all ways of healing have one precept common: To heal is to make whole, and healing means *restoring wholeness*.

The word 'health' comes from the word *hale*, meaning whole, hence the term (w)holistic medicine. Lack of health implies disintegration, loss of balance, disorder of the fine-tuning of mental, spiritual and bodily functions. Symptoms are messages that things are not flowing smoothly within us. Many drugs just suppress these important messages, whereas most non-drug therapies seek to correct the underlying imbalance by helping the body to restore its own wholeness.

There is of course a lot of overlap between modern Western medicine and the so-called 'alternative' therapies. The visit to a doctor who also has a gift for healing (which is not given to all, in spite of degrees, diplomas, and modern technology) is in itself therapeutic.

You tell your complete story to someone who is prepared to listen. You receive words of explanation and comfort, and the touch of healing hands through a handshake or examination. You may be given a prescription for a medicine, and you are encouraged to *believe* that it will help you. The patient's belief that something will do good is an important part of any therapy, whether it is a bottle of pills, herbs, acupuncture, or manipulation. This is called the *placebo effect*. It is natural and valid in all forms of healing, whether the healer is a witch-doctor, a famous specialist, a family doctor or a herbalist.

The patient's belief in the possibility of improvement is a significant part of any healing therapy, because of the influence that mental attitude has over bodily recovery. It is known that among people with a serious illness, such as cancer, those who have an optimistic outlook, and a reason for staying alive, tend to do better than those who are pessimists and feel helpless.

M.E. sufferers who get better report a great range of reasons for their recovery. In all survey questionnaires asking 'What things have helped you?', top of the league is *rest*. A variety of other therapies are mentioned, including changing one's diet, homoeopathy, gentle exercise, taking evening primrose oil, painkillers, anti-depressants, and treating Candida; some people have improved after the laying on of hands in Christian healing. So far, there is no single treatment that cures M.E. and CFS, whether it be a drug, diet, or a complementary therapy.

It cannot be repeated too often that *you need to rest, whatever else you undertake in the search for healing*. The energy expenditure involved in travelling long distances to find a therapist who will cure you may undo the benefits of the treatment.

Homoeopathy

The word 'homoeopathy' comes from two Greek words, *homois* and *pathos*, meaning *similar* and *suffering* respectively.

A homoeopathic remedy is a specially diluted preparation of a substance which, when taken by a healthy person, produces a symptom picture that is similar to that of the patient. Homoeopathy follows the principle of 'like treats like', unlike allopathic, Western medicine, which treats symptoms with substances having opposite effects.

An example of homoeopathic medicine which was actually used as a conventional drug is quinine. This is derived from the bark of a tree, which if taken over some time produces symptoms of shivering, sweating, and fever. A weaker extract of this tree bark is prepared as the drug quinine, and was used to treat malaria.

A homoeopathic remedy is prepared by diluting the medicine many times, in a process of serial dilutions called 'potentization'. In the resulting dilution there may be few or no molecules of the original substance left; however, during the dilution process the mixture is shaken very vigorously at each stage, and it is thought that some biologically active property (perhaps an electrical one?) of the molecules of the original drug is imparted to the resulting potentized remedy, whether the dilution is effected with a liquid or a solid.

The weaker the concentration of a remedy, the more highly potentized it is, and the more powerful it is in its curative effect. This is one of the stumbling blocks for scientifically-minded doctors in accepting homoeopathy. The curative effect seems to be from gentle stimulation of the body to rid itself of whatever is causing the symptoms.

A homoeopathic remedy is selected after a careful history-taking, to establish not only all the patient's symptoms, but other characteristics such as personality, seasonal influence, food habits, and any other factors that influence symptoms. So no one remedy is prescribed for any one symptom; three patients with rheumatism may each require a different remedy, according to the total symptom and character picture of each of them.

Good homoeopathic prescribing requires skill and experience, and it is best to consult a fully-trained practitioner. Homoeopathy is safe: even if the wrong remedy is prescribed, no harm results. However, when treating a chronic condition, it is common to have temporary worsening of symptoms to start with. Some remedies are used to treat symptoms only, and can be bought and self-prescribed for first aid and home use. These are in low potencies, and are very useful for first-aid treatment of such things as headache, fever, stomach upsets, etc. For example, Arnica 6c is a remedy for bruising, sprains, and muscle pain due to overuse.

To treat a chronic condition, a higher potency may be used, and fewer doses are taken. The deepest level of homoeopathic treatment for M.E. is given by identifying the infection which is persisting in the body and causing symptoms, then giving a homoeopathic preparation of the original virus that started the illness. This type of remedy is called a *nosode*. Nosodes of chronic infections thought to be the past origins of ill health have been used in homoeopathy for a long time, for example Tuberculinum.

A virus nosode used to treat M.E. may be not the exact virus but may be of its family. It is possible to make a homoeopathic preparation of any infective agent.

There are two difficulties about this homoeopathic approach to M.E. The first is identifying the culprit that needs to be treated. The second is that if the correct nosode is taken, it is likely to induce a temporary revival of all the original symptoms of the infection that triggered off the M.E. syndrome. However, the apparent severe relapse should not last very long, a few days to a few weeks, and should be seen as a good thing, a sign that the correct remedy has been chosen and the body is being stimulated to get rid of the persisting infection.

Some remedies that have been mentioned by various M.E. patients as being helpful include:

- Aconite – for great fear and anxiety, especially at night, for the 'feeling of dying', with pressure on the chest, breathing difficulty, or fluttering heart
- Sepia – for dragging weariness (in women), premenstrual symptoms, and with loss of feeling for loved ones

- Arnica – for aching muscles and joints, or exhaustion from overdoing things
- Bryonia – for arthritic pain, bursting headache, all pains that are better for pressure, and for lack of movement

Polio Nosode

A homoeopathic practitioner has used a nosode from poliovirus to treat some M.E. patients:

> I give single doses of increasing potencies at 8-hour intervals (as one single potency causes too severe aggravation). This still gives a bit of a knock for 24 hours, but patients sit up, get moving and feel much better. The Polio is repeated when the muscle weakness starts to come back, which will be less and less frequently.
>
> *(Personal communication from Dr B. Boss, Johannesburg)*

I know one M.E. patient whose illness dates from becoming ill during a local polio outbreak during 1955 when she was 15 – the same year as the M.E. outbreaks in the Royal Free and Durban hospitals. She has been greatly strengthened by having homoeopathic polio prescribed by the above-quoted practitioner.

For further information and advice about the value of homoeopathy, you are advised to read one of the several excellent books available (one is listed at the end of this chapter), or to consult a qualified practitioner.

Acupuncture

Many people think of acupuncture as being mainly a treatment for pain. This healing art has been used by the Chinese for thousands of years, not only to treat pain but all kinds of illness, and also to maintain health.

A Chinese physician does not diagnose in the same way as his or her Western counterpart would. History and examination are carried out, but with particular attention to the appearance of the patient's face and tongue, and the quality of the pulse at both wrists. The practitioner is looking for signs of an imbalance of body energies, and of how the body functions are disturbed.

There is no such diagnosis as M.E. in Chinese medicine. A patient who presents with complaints of exhaustion, muscle weakness, feeling cold and insomnia would be diagnosed as suffering from deficient *Chi* (energy), and deficiency of Chi in various organs such as the heart, spleen and liver. Another patient may have a slightly different diagnosis, but all M.E. sufferers are basically lacking in body energy; this is reflected in poor function of the organs, cold, and stagnation of Chi in energy pathways, leading to pain, poor digestion and absorption of food, or disturbed mental function.

Chinese medicine pays attention to the lifestyle of the patient, and advises on changing it where appropriate. M.E. and CFS would be regarded as conditions where the patient had depleted his or her energy and had no defence against bodily invasion of a pathogenic factor, which would not be expelled but would go deep into the body and upset the workings of vital organs. Substitute 'virus' for 'pathogenic factor' and you have a good account of the development of M.E.

Acupuncture treatment for M.E. needs to be given in a way that does not drain energy from the patient, but rather supplies energy, or else stimulates the body's immune system. A technique that supplies energy is to use a burning herb (moxa) over acupuncture points, the warmth entering the energy channels and dispersing cold, and invigorating body organs. The smouldering moxa does not burn the skin, it only creates a sensation of heat.

There is no single prescription in Chinese medicine for treating M.E. Each patient is assessed individually, and a diagnosis is formulated which may vary in different systems of Chinese teaching. In China, herbs are used with or without acupuncture.

It is important to consult a fully-trained practitioner,

rather than someone who has only done a weekend course, and only knows how to treat pain. An unskilled acupuncturist may make an M.E. patient worse, by giving treatment in a way that results in energy being drained away. For M.E., acupuncture treatment needs to be gentle, and to be given in a way that does *not remove energy*. Most M.E. patients are extremely sensitive, and may have a greater reaction to acupuncture than other people.

The insertion of an acupuncture needle is swift and virtually painless. If the needle is then manipulated there is a sensation which varies from a deep ache to a tingling or a numbness – this indicates that the point has been correctly located and the needle will do its work. Few patients complain of pain from acupuncture therapy, and if any is felt, it is short-lived.

On the whole, acupuncture needling is not appropriate for someone in a severe stage of M.E., nor for patients who are very sensitive with a lot of muscle pain. Moxa (heat) treatment is more acceptable in such cases. Some therapists now use a laser which stimulates the energy point below the skin, instead of needles. All properly trained practitioners are scrupulous about needle sterility, and most now use disposable needles.

Acupuncture can be helpful for insomnia, muscle pain, nervous symptoms and digestive problems in M.E. and CFS.

Massage and Aromatherapy

Many people find massage helpful. If you cannot find a trained therapist locally, or cannot go out for treatment, look for a book which instructs simple massage techniques for a carer to learn. The massage needs to be extremely gentle, especially if the patient is very ill or has a lot of body pain. There is no place for the vigorous pummelling and rubbing traditionally thought of as massage.

Much of the benefit of massage comes from the physical touch of a caring person, just as a mother soothes a child by stroking its head. The emphasis should be on comforting, soothing, and relaxing rather than on trying to massage away muscle pain. The body is so sensitive in M.E. that a much lighter touch is needed than in massage for a fit person.

Aromatherapy is given by a practitioner who is trained in massage and also uses essential oils on the skin for their therapeutic properties. After an initial consultation, an aromatherapist may give you a supply of the oils he or she has used, for you to rub in yourself at home, or to add to the bath. The prescription used will be individual to your needs, based on your symptoms. The oils are pure extracts from various plants which have healing properties, known for centuries. They do not contain colourings or chemicals; minute amounts are absorbed through the skin and fragrance is inhaled to produce beneficial effects.

Essential oils work on one level by relieving stress and anxiety; at a deeper level they can balance body energies and benefit the immune system. Different oils are used for different emotional and physical problems; some have stimulating properties (such as eucalyptus), others are relaxing and sedating (such as sandalwood), others affect functions such as digestion and hormone levels. *Stimulating oils should not be used on people with M.E.*

Those who have tried aromatherapy have found it very pleasant, and comforting. Benefits include muscle relaxation, less muscle pain, better sleep and less anxiety. If a practitioner can be found who can visit you at home, so much the better.

Bach Flower Remedies

Bach Remedies are made from various different plants, each of which has a specific effect on a disordered emotional state. They are different from herbal preparations, in that they are very dilute pure preparations and work exclusively on the emotions rather than on other bodily symptoms. They are absolutely safe, and if a remedy is chosen which is inappropriate for the emotional state, there is no harmful effect.

The most useful to keep at hand is Bach's Rescue Remedy, which is made from five specific remedies, and can be used in a situation of sudden mental shock or collapse. Another useful remedy is Olive, which helps a fatigued, exhausted mind.

Herbal Medicines

Plants with specific healing properties have been used to prepare medicines, poultices, powders, etc. for a very long time, throughout the world. Some of our modern drugs are derived from plant medicines: for example Digoxin, used for heart failure, is a synthetic form of digitalis, obtained from the leaves of the foxglove.

On the whole, herbal medicines are safer than modern, synthetic drugs, so long as they are taken in the prescribed way. A qualified medical herbalist does five years of training that includes anatomy, physiology, and study of illness (pathology), as well as learning a vast amount about botany and the pharmacology of plants. For first-aid use at home, herbal remedies are available in herbalists, many pharmacists and health food shops; these medicines are all safe if used correctly.

For treatment of chronic ailments and deep-seated symptoms, it is best to consult a qualified herbalist – who will take a detailed history, and prescribe a herb, or more usually, a combination of herbs, not just to suppress symptoms but to help correct the cause of illness. Chinese medicine uses herbs as much as acupuncture, and there are many similarities in diagnosis and prescription between Chinese herbal medicine, and herbal medicine as instructed in Western countries.

The property of a plant for healing purposes is not classified as being 'good for cough' (for example), but rather in terms of its functions of heating or cooling, stimulating or sedating, contracting or relaxing of smooth muscle, antiseptic, blood purifying, etc. Some are particularly rich in essential minerals, which may be depleted in disease.

Some of the commonest herbs are found in our gardens and kitchens, such as onion, garlic, parsley, thyme, mint, sage, ginger, and cayenne. Many familiar garden plants have powerful properties, including nettles, dandelions, and marigold.

Many herbal preparations have side-effects *if used incorrectly* or if the wrong part of a plant is used, but the toxic side-effects are rare in comparison with side-effects from synthetic chemical drugs.

There are certain herbs that have anti-viral properties. One of these is *Hydrastis Canadensis* – commonly known as Golden Seal. Another is *Allium sativum* – which is garlic, well known as an anti-infection plant.

Several herbs are being investigated in the USA, and are known to have immune-stimulating properties (they have been used in treatment for HIV/AIDS with some success). These are: *Echinacea*, *Lomatium*, and an extract from Shiitake.

Shiitake is a Chinese medicinal mushroom which has been used for centuries to stimulate the immune system. 'The extract is called LEM, and has been found to increases the number of total white cells, T-cells, and has antiviral properties' (CFIDS Physician's Forum, March 1991). At the time of writing, I do not know if LEM is available in the UK.

Herbal teas are alternatives to tea or coffee. There are a good variety available now. It is helpful to know their different properties – for example, peppermint aids digestion, and chamomile is a natural sedative and suitable for the evening.

Yoga and T'ai Chi are both therapies and exercise. They

have been discussed in Chapter 8.

Natural Healing

Healing by the laying on of hands, and through prayer, has been around for a long time. Some people are born with a special gift of healing. They can transmit healing energy to a sick person through their hands, and with the same hands can tell what parts of the body are not functioning properly. Some professional healers use purely physical healing energy, others use a spiritual approach as well as physical. The latter may have had teaching from the National Federation of Spiritual Healing (address in Appendix A). Most spiritual healers offer their services free, and accept whatever payment the patient wishes and is able to give.

I personally believe that regular prayer by a number of people does bring about healing in the sick person prayed for, even if the recipient does not profess any religious faith. Healing by prayer or by touch cannot be measured scientifically. This is a good thing; we need to accept some 'miracles' in our mechanized, material world. We also need to accept that there are many mysteries in life. Wisdom comes with acceptance of, and belief in, mystery and miracles as well as scientific facts.

Two other natural therapies that are freely available and cost nothing are daylight and fresh air.

Natural Light

Natural daylight and sunshine are extremely important for health because:

the skin makes vitamin D in daylight
full-spectrum light entering the eyes has a direct effect
    on health
they give one a psychological boost.

Various behavioural patterns in animals and plants –

such as growth, courtship and breeding, migration, hibernation, sleep and activity, the opening of flowers – result from changes in light.

Light exerts a profound effect on plants and all animal life. We humans have largely overcome the lifestyle restrictions once enforced by darkness through the invention of electric light. Oil lamps, candles and gas lamps did not influence our way of life to the extent that electricity has. With electric light, people can stay awake as late as they like, can work all day without daylight, sit up late watching TV, and play football at night. We have lost the habit of sleeping more in winter than in summer, and maybe this is why peoples' energy levels and resistance to infection are depleted in late winter and early spring.

Dr John Ott, an American scientist, studied the effects of different kinds of light on plants, animals and humans in the 1960s and 1970s. In his book *Health and Light* he describes the difference in the health and size of some animals in breeding sheds, where one shed received more reflected light than the other. The animals that had more light were healthier, larger, and had more offspring than those in sheds where light was poor. Other factors – food, temperature, and cage size – were identical. Dr Ott (using a UV light meter) found decidedly higher levels of ultraviolet light being reflected into the areas where the animals had been doing very well.

Dr Ott, talking of the loss of light from air pollution in cities, says:

. . . civilized man has cut himself off from more sunlight by living indoors behind walls and glass. Man has developed artificial sources of illumination that have almost no ultraviolet and distort the light spectrum of natural sunlight. More people wear glasses or contact lenses, which cut down ultraviolet light entering the eyes. To what extent is this polluted light environment affecting man's health and well-being?

John Ott also records how he himself suffered badly from arthritis, at a time when he was spending a lot of time inside, making time-sequence movie shots of plants. He accidentally broke his glasses, and spent some days outside in sunlight, being unable to drive or to work without them. To his surprise, his arthritic pains improved dramatically, but worsened if he had to spend time again inside or behind glass. He had previously rested lying in sunlight, wearing sunglasses, with no benefit to the arthritis at all. He found that the pain eased only when he exposed his eyes (without wearing his glasses) to full-spectrum light for several hours a day.

The mechanism whereby exposure to full-spectrum daylight affects mood, health and animal fertility is not fully investigated. The influence of light depends largely on an adequate level of the ultraviolet part of visible light being received in the eyes. There are direct nerve connections between photoreceptive cells in the eye and the pineal gland, which is a small outgrowth of the brain situated behind the hypothalamus, deep within the brain.

The pineal is probably involved in co-ordinating circadian and diurnal rhythms in different organs of the body, doing this by way of the hypothalamus and pituitary gland. It seems to be an active gland, and may secrete hormones into the circulation to affect other parts of the body; so it could influence general health, probably via other hormone-secreting glands.

Many M.E. sufferers deteriorate from November through till the spring. Maybe lack of light is responsible, as well as winter cold and damp, and increased indoor pollution.

In tuberculosis sanatoria, in the days before drugs for treating TB came into being, ill patients on long-term rest were put outside on open verandas all the year round, so they could receive the benefits of both fresh air and sunlight.

I am not suggesting that people with M.E., who are

frequently light-sensitive, should sit outside and stare at the sun. But it does make sense to get outside each day if you are well enough; in strong sunlight rest in the shade, for there is still plenty of reflected full-spectrum light. Someone virtually bedridden should at least spend some time by a window; even though glass cuts out some light, it is better than nothing. If you wear glasses, leave them off while sitting or resting outside. Light enters even through closed eyelids. If you cannot get outside much, get a full-spectrum light-bulb, and use it in the room where you spend most of your day. These lamps are supplied by some garden centres (for winter plants) and also by some health shops.

Fresh Air and Oxygen

Unpolluted air is desirable for everyone. Oxygen is essential, but there are many unwanted substances in the air that damage lungs, affect children's brains (especially lead from car exhausts), and make chemically-sensitive people ill. Fortunately the air in most cities in the UK has improved in quality following the Clean Air Act and the introduction of smoke-free zones. But the visible smoke and smog from thousands of coal fires has been replaced by ever-increasing pollution from petrol and diesel fumes, as more and more people use cars instead of their feet or public transport.

Pollution is just as bad *inside* many buildings, because of the increased use of plastic and foam-based furnishings and equipment, air conditioning which may recirculate dust and germs, sprays and air 'fresheners'.

The oxygen supply of some tissues in M.E. seems to be poor, especially during a relapse. There are several possible reasons for this. The first is the abnormal shape of some red cells (see page 63) and disordered regulation of circulation by the brain control centre that seems to accompany M.E. M.E. also seems to cause some disorder of breathing regulation, especially at night. Tests on M.E. patients in a sleep laboratory have shown that there are periods during sleep when a patient stops breathing for a minute or so – these are called 'apnoea' periods. This may explain the alarming symptom of waking up feeling short of breath, and needing to sit up and take deep breaths.

Preliminary trials of oxygen therapy to M.E. patients have shown some benefit. The procedure is to supply oxygen via a small nasal tube during sleep. For those who are very ill, especially with symptoms of bad circulation or evidence of poor oxygenation of the tissues, it may be possible to have an oxygen supply on loan from the NHS, to use at night; the oxygen is dispensed through a nasal catheter.

It is a good idea, even if house-bound, to do some deep breathing daily beside an open window. Breathing exercises can be learned from relaxation tapes, or from Yoga teaching. In modern centrally-heated double-glazed homes, ventilation is often poor, allowing build-up of moulds and dust. So each room should be properly aired each day by opening a window for a time (see Chapter 15 for more ideas on keeping the air in your home as fresh as possible).

Hyperbaric Oxygen Therapy

Hyperbaric oxygen therapy may be of benefit to some M.E. sufferers. The treatment involves breathing oxygen under pressure, sitting in a large chamber alongside other patients. This results in an increased oxygen-partial pressure in the blood, with improved delivery of oxygen to all tissues.

Hyperbaric oxygen therapy has been used for some years by people with Multiple Sclerosis. Treatment chambers are available at various ARMS (Action for Research into Multiple Sclerosis) treatment centres around the UK.

In theory it should be helpful for the many symptoms

of M.E. that are associated with poor oxygenation of tissues and problems of cell membrane function, such as muscle pains, poor brain function, and low energy levels. It is unlikely to hasten the departure of a persistent virus. It is hoped that more will be learned about this therapy and M.E. in due course.

A doctor attached to ARMS has reported symptomatic improvement in 28 out of 36 patients (diagnosed elsewhere as M.E.) attending a HBO therapy centre (Perrins, 1990).

Meanwhile, M.E. sufferers wishing to find out more about hyperbaric oxygen therapy and location of treatment centres should contact ARMS (address given in Appendix A).

There are of course many other therapies that have not been mentioned here; this is not because they are unknown or useless. Those described in this chapter have all been helpful to some M.E. sufferers. It appears that homoeopathy has helped more people than the other therapies have, but in the absence of any organized treatment trials, evidence of one treatment being better than another can only be based on anecdotal evidence.

Suggested Further Reading

Homoeopathy: A Family Handbook, (Thorsons, 1992).
Robert Tisserand, *Aromatherapy for Everyone*, (Penguin, 1988).
Barbara Griggs, *The Home Herbal*, (Pan, 1986).

Chapter 18

Women with M.E.

Women seem to be affected by M.E. about three times as often as men in the age group 20–50, the years of both employment and fertility. Of course, in institutions where outbreaks occur, e.g. an army camp, or a nurses' residential home, there may be 100 per cent of the men or women affected. Yet, because of what seems to be M.E.'s 'bias' towards women, some doctors wrongly conclude that hysteria and neurosis contribute to the disease. This is inaccurate, speculative and scientifically unproven rubbish, and is insulting to women. This attitude continues to prevail, however, mainly among paternalistic older male doctors.

In fact, the reasons for the female/male ratio in M.E. are simple, if one accepts that the illness is virus triggered, often in people who are stressed or exhausted: Who are the people most exposed to viruses, particularly enteroviruses? Who are the people most likely to have to carry on working even when they are ill with a virus infection, or to have to return to work before properly recovered?

The high-risk occupations for contact with enteroviruses are:

1. Teachers, especially of primary school.
2. Mothers, many of whom hold two jobs – homemaker plus outside paid work.
3. Nurses and those in other health care jobs.
4. Agricultural and sewage workers (yes, these are usually men).
5. To some extent, all jobs with high levels of public

contact expose the worker to more viruses.

Of these, the people least likely to be able to rest enough from a viral infection are mothers of young children, teachers, and all health care workers, particularly nurses. A man with an office job, not coming into contact with a lot of children, who can sign off work for a week and be cared for at home if he gets flu, is probably at lower risk of M.E. This is not sexist propaganda, just commonsense observation!

There may also be a hormonal link with the conditions in the body that are right for M.E. to develop, but the mechanisms of this are not established. It may just be coincidence that the child-bearing years (18–40) are also the years of maximum hard work in high-risk jobs.

Problems Particular to Women with M.E.

Menstrual periods – painful, irregular, heavy, or disappearing altogether.
Endometriosis
Premenstrual syndrome (often called PMT), which may become worse with M.E.
Pregnancy – to be or not? Will the baby be affected?
Contraception – is the pill OK?
Menopause plus M.E. – may make each other worse
Cystitis
Vaginal infections
Relationships and sex
Not every woman who gets M.E. will have problems in any of these areas. And of course a lot of women who do not have M.E. suffer from these gynaecological problems, but they may be much worse after developing this illness.

Periods
In some women, their cycle may become longer, shorter or irregular. Periods may be lighter or heavier than

before, or even disappear during severe illness. These changes may happen with any long-term illness, also with chronic stress.

If periods become heavier, then extra iron and vitamin C are indicated. There is sometimes a disturbance of thyroid function with M.E., and this may be associated with prolonged flow.

Tampons are better *not* used during a period, because of the increased risk of vaginal infection.

Endometriosis

There are a significant number of women who suffer from an unpleasant gynaecological condition called endometriosis, as well as having M.E. In endometriosis, tiny pieces of endometrium (the lining of the womb, which is shed with every period), grow outside the womb. These abnormally situated endometrial tissues can be found anywhere, mostly lying on the outer surface of the womb, on the bladder, on the large bowel, or the ovaries and their supporting tissues. These 'seeded' tissues grow and then bleed at each period, and cause a lot of pain, and also scar tissue.

Typical symptoms are:

- Severe period pain
- Deep pelvic pain during and after intercourse
- Unexplained lower abdominal and pelvic pain, any time in the cycle
- Infertility
- Irregular bleeding or bleeding from other sites, such as the bladder or rectum

The condition can only be diagnosed with certainty by surgery or laparoscopy. The cause of endometriosis is not understood. It can affect women at any age from puberty up till the onset of the menopause. There appears to be an association with Candidiasis, and current research is finding abnormal immune functions similar to those in M.E. It is possible that a common mechanism predisposes a woman to having both endometriosis and M.E.

Current treatment for endometriosis is either hormonal – something to suppress oestrogen levels – or surgical. The latter involves removing affected tissues, often including the ovary and Fallopian tube, or a hysterectomy. For a lot of women with this condition, a big problem is getting their doctor to recognize it; he or she may instead dismiss their increasingly severe menstrual and pelvic pain as psychological, and refuse to refer for a specialist opinion.

Endometriosis sufferers with M.E. need to be cautious about hormone therapy, which might cause a severe M.E. relapse in some cases. High dose essential fatty acids (such as evening primrose oil, see page 166), B vitamins, magnesium, and anti-Candida treatment may be worth trying before agreeing to more drastic treatment.

I have described endometriosis in some detail, because of the increasing evidence that the condition may be more common in M.E. than in non-M.E. women, and because anti-Candida approaches may help (see Chapter 13). Some women with M.E. may attribute all pelvic symptoms to the M.E., and not seek help and further diagnosis – another reminder that when you have M.E., you must not assume all new symptoms are caused by it – especially pain, which may be due to something else and may be treatable.

In the UK (and USA) there is a 'M.E. and Endo' support group, which can provide support and further information (it can be contacted through M.E. Action – address in Appendix A)

Premenstrual Syndrome

Also commonly known as PMT – premenstrual tension, though tension is not the only symptom, but only the one most obvious to other people! Premenstrual syndrome means that symptoms appear only during the

10 days before a period and are relieved when the period starts. Common symptoms are:

- weight gain
- bloating
- tender, swollen breasts
- irritability
- irrational behaviour
- depression
- weeping
- mood swings
- insomnia
- food cravings (usually for sugar and chocolate)
- headaches.

Many of these symptoms are due to fluid retention, and overlap with Candidiasis (which may contribute to PMS). If the condition has been experienced before M.E., then it may become worse once you have M.E. as well.

Measures to Improve PMS
Avoid blood-sugar swings by having small, frequent meals of complex carbohydrates regularly, and forgoing sugar and red meats. Stimulants such as coffee and tea should be reduced. Salt intake should be cut down.

The following supplements are of proven value:

- Gamma linoleic acid as evening primrose oil (EPO): at least 2 gm daily. If EPO is being taken to help M.E. it is a good idea to increase the dose during the premenstrual time.
- Magnesium: 250–500 mg a day
- Vitamin B_6: 50 mg a day in addition to B vitamins taken as part of a good multivitamin preparation. (See address of Women's Nutritional Advisory Service in Appendix A).
- The homoeopathic remedy Sepia is useful for symptoms of exhaustion, weariness, and depression.

It is also important to be aware of any reduced mental function or emotional control at this time, and to avoid tasks involving important decisions, and situations you know from experience will bring out your worst side. (I try to avoid driving if PMT is bad, for fear of hitting other cars in rage or impatience!)

If the PMS is severe and the subject is over 40, it may be worth asking for hormone assessment from a doctor. I know two women who suffer from M.E. plus severe PMS depression, who have been helped by hormone therapy (commonly a small dose of progesterone). It may seem strange that I mention this, in apparent contradiction to my advice against taking the contraceptive pill in Chapter 16, and below. However, no treatment is 'black and white' with M.E. It is important to remember that other treatable medical conditions, in this case menopausal premenstrual depression (which can be devastating in M.E.), may need to be diagnosed and treated with conventional treatment.

Most of the symptoms of PMS are probably due to water-retention. This mechanism also happens in M.E., apart from PMS, and contributes to weight gain, headaches and other brain symptoms (see page 70).

Pregnancy

No doubt quite a number of women who have M.E. have successful pregnancies. Advice is commonly given from patient support groups that M.E. will not harm the baby. No one denies that there will be extra fatigue during the early years of caring for babies and young children. However, the most serious questions in the minds of women who have diagnosed M.E. and wish to have a baby, are these:

What chance is there that my illness could harm the baby? Can M.E. be passed on to a young child? Will my husband and I be able to cope with the extra demands of pregnancy, labour, and sleep loss after the birth?

There are no simple answers to these questions. Early

research has found a small but definite number of M.E. pregnancies that have not progressed normally.

Any virus, if active during early pregnancy, may occasionally cause miscarriage, or abnormalities in the newborn. Rubella (German measles virus) and cytomegalovirus are well-known culprits. In a 35-year follow-up of family contacts of proven cases of enterovirus infection (in one area of England), Dr John Richardson, general practitioner, estimated a foetal loss of 30 per cent (of which at least 5 per cent is natural loss). This includes miscarriage, stillbirth and congenital abnormalities. (Personal communication from Dr E. Dowsett.)

There is also the probability that there is some inherited factor which may make the child more susceptible to M.E. – in the same way that a tendency to allergies is inherited (and seems to be more common among relatives of M.E. sufferers). In this way a mother may pass on a gene that makes the child vulnerable to getting M.E. Further research may clarify this potential hazard of childbearing. Any inherited susceptibility to M.E. applies, of course, to fathers as well as mothers.

Some M.E. women feel better throughout pregnancy (which is a natural immune suppressant), but relapse after an exhausting birth, or with the post-natal drop in hormones. Some are ill throughout pregnancy. The consensus of advice from doctors, and from mothers who have experience of M.E., is to put off pregnancy until the M.E. has stabilized and signs suggesting infection (e.g. fevers, diarrhoea, lymph glands, throat infections) are settled.

Then, only consider it if the mum-to-be can rest well during pregnancy, and if plenty of domestic help is planned (and budgeted for – more important than fancy frills for the baby) after the birth. I have not heard of any evidence to show that breast-feeding passes on M.E. to an infant. Breast-milk, if available, will provide the best protection against other infection, and also the best source of natural GLA (an essential fatty acid) to protect the infant against developing allergies. Obviously good nutrition is supremely important during pregnancy and while breast-feeding. A useful source of information on nutrition for pregnancy, especially for women with allergies, chronic infections or a history of pregnancy disasters of any kind, is the organization Foresight (address in Appendix A).

Even the strongest of new mothers can suffer from post-natal depression, lack of sleep, and exhaustion. M.E. will not exempt you from these tribulations! However, the joy of a new child may well outweigh the problems, and a decision about embarking on a pregnancy must be yours and your partner's.

Childbirth
The question of drugs during labour, such as painkillers, gas and air, or an epidural, is one to discuss beforehand with your obstetrician and midwife. Many women with M.E. do cope quite well with labour, however exhaustion in the second stage may set in earlier than normal, so that there may be a greater likelihood of needing help (e.g. forceps) with delivery. It is wise to let the health workers concerned with your pregnancy and delivery know in advance about M.E. and how it affects you, emphasizing the nature of the muscle fatigability.

Contraception
This is obviously important if pregnancy is thought to be a potential hazard, and should be discussed with your GP or a family planning clinic. The pill has many drawbacks even for non-M.E. women:

- increases the likelihood of Candida infections
- reduces the available levels of vitamin B_6
- increases the likelihood of depression
- interferes with carbohydrate metabolism.
- Zinc deficiency is associated with taking the pill.

- The pill has been shown to affect the function of the immune system.
- Women who have taken the pill for some years have increased incidence of allergies and immune dysfunction diseases.

It is probably safer to avoid the contraceptive pill if you have M.E., for all the above reasons, and also because female hormones are related to steroids and might in theory have adverse effects on the body's own steroid production and interfere with natural immunity.

Intrauterine devices – 'coils' – can lead to infection in the womb and heavy periods, complications anyone with M.E. would wish to avoid. The safest birth control would be to use the barrier methods: A diaphragm or cervical cap plus spermicidal cream. Or a combination of a condom plus spermicidal cream.

The alternative, if you and your partner are sure you do not want any children in the future, is sterilization – tubal ligation in the woman or vasectomy for the man. These methods are virtually 100 per cent effective for birth control, but are final, and couples need careful counselling before making this decision.

Menopause

There is nothing you can do stop the passage of time if you are over 40. The change of life is a fact of life. In many women this time is passed uneventfully, but others experience distressing symptoms, which may be confused with chronic fatigue syndrome by those without clear knowledge of CFS or M.E. These are:

- abnormal fatigue
- mood swings
- depression
- sweatings
- flushings.

Anyone familiar with the true features of M.E. will be

able to distinguish M.E. from the menopause, as the former has the particular muscle fatigability, and symptoms made worse by exercise – not the same as the general weariness and slowing down of a woman during the menopause. The problem the menopause poses with M.E. is that one seems to make the other worse. Also, menopausal women with severe symptoms, especially of fatigue, may wrongly fear that they have M.E. This makes diagnosis and exclusion of other conditions especially important for the self-diagnosed sufferer at this age. If M.E. is already diagnosed and pre-exists, the onset of the menopause may exacerbate some symptoms. Any major life change is a stress on the body, including puberty and the menopause. If M.E. depression is much worse at this time, consider asking your doctor if hormone therapy might help (see above in section on PMS).

Cystitis

This bladder problem is not confined to women, but seems to be more common among them. Symptoms of frequency of, urgency of, or burning on passing water, blood in urine (if severe), lower abdominal pain, and fever, suggest infection in the bladder.

Management

Drink masses of water, rest completely, and see your doctor as soon as possible so that a urine specimen can be collected in a special bottle for bacteriological testing. A simple remedy, obtainable from any pharmacy, is potassium citrate (Mist Pot Cit), which makes urine more alkaline and reduces the burning.

If the symptoms are not severe, it is better to wait until results of the urine culture before starting antibiotics. Then, if no bacterial infection is found, you will not have unnecessary antibiotics (a bad thing with M.E.), and if infection is present, the drug sensitivities will be found and the correct antibiotic prescribed.

What happens sometimes is that all the nasty symptoms of a bladder infection are present, but no bugs are found in the urine. It is possible in such cases that:

the infection is a yeast one (Candida)
food allergies are another possible culprit
there is some disturbance of bladder sensation and bladder function, locally or maybe centrally in the brain.

Anyone who has repeated attacks of cystitis should make sure her nutrition is good and take extra supplements to boost resistance to infection.

Some herbs are helpful for bladder symptoms, e.g. Potter's 'Antitis tablets' and Marshmallow root.

The homoeopathic remedy for acute symptoms is usually Cantharis.

However, if you have an acute attack of cystitis, you must see a doctor and have any bacterial infection identified and treated. Untreated bacterial bladder infections can spread to the kidneys and cause serious problems – with or without M.E.

Vaginal Infections

Recurrent thrush is a common female problem made worse with M.E. However, any abnormal discharge should be investigated if it persists. It may indicate some other infection which needs treatment. Thrush, caused by the yeast Candida Albicans, typically causes a white discharge, with intense itching around the vaginal entrance. If the discharge is yellow, offensive or blood-stained, you must see your doctor. Thrush tends to flare up in conditions of poor health, stress, too much sugar in the diet, diabetes, taking birth control pills, local conditions of heat and humidity (e.g. wearing nylon tights and pants, or in hot humid weather) and poor hygiene.

General anti-Candida measures will help (see Chapter 13), plus treatment with vaginal pessaries and cream.

The latter alone will not clear up thrush for long if your diet is wrong. As the bugs causing vaginal infections are transmitted to and from a sexual partner, it is better to abstain from sex while the infection lasts, and it is best for your partner to get treated as well. Another common bug is Trichomonas, which like Candida is widespread and easily transferred between partners.

The use of tampons during a period may increase the likelihood of vaginal infection, as they act as a reservoir of blood in which bugs multiply, especially if not changed regularly. There are recorded cases where a forgotten tampon has led to a very severe infection which has spread to the bloodstream. While the majority of non-M.E. women can happily use tampons all their lives with no complications, I believe that if you have M.E. it is prudent to minimize risks of any infection in the body.

Sexual Relationships

The problems sexual relationships (or rather the lack of them!) cause with M.E. are discussed more fully in Chapter 21. Loss of interest in sex is a very common symptom for both men and women with M.E. and any chronic fatigue syndrome. The body wishes to use available energy for what it considers more important activities. Loss of interest in sex is also a common symptom in severe depression, low thyroid function, and many other chronic illnesses. If depression is a prominent complication of M.E., treatment of this by antidepressants or counselling might improve an M.E. person's sex life somewhat.

Even if always exhausted, a wise woman will try and find times when sex is least stressful, to reassure a caring partner that he is still loved and needed. As with post-menopausal women, vaginal dryness and discomfort may be discouraging, but using KY lubricating jelly may sometimes help.

Loss of an adequate sex life (every couple has different needs) can be very detrimental to a relationship already rocked by the effects of illness on one and perhaps both partners. Sometimes there are psychological blocks as well as physical constraints, and some time with a skilled counsellor may help one or both partners (the organization Sexual Problems of Disabled People (SPOD) may be helpful – address in Appendix A).

Chapter 19

Finance and Practical Problems

It is bad enough to have a disabling disease that causes pain and exhaustion, but many people with M.E. endure the added stress of financial hardship, through being unable to work. Many are highly motivated, hard-working, self-reliant people, to whom the idea of accepting State benefit may have been unthinkable before natural retirement.

Employment and State Benefits in the UK

When you first become ill you may be in an employed position, and therefore eligible for sick pay. If you are self-employed, you may be able to get Sickness Benefit.

The real problems arise if you are still ill after six months (28 weeks), at which point you and everyone else start to wonder how long this is going to go on for. If you are making some recovery it may be tempting to try going back to work. If the job is full-time, and physically and emotionally demanding – such as nursing, or teaching – the chances are that you quickly find out that you are *not* fully recovered, have to stop work again, and have a major relapse brought on by the exertion. No one can predict at this stage if you will need a further six months off, or a year, or more.

You must accept that *your health comes first*, and if you need more time completely off work, that is what has to happen. Some people may be able to negotiate part-time work, with the flexibility of going home or resting should their energy run out. But these kinds of jobs are rare. When considering whether or not to stop work completely, you need to ask yourself if the job is going to hinder further recovery, or if you can manage to improve despite the job.

It may turn out to be possible to work, but only if a lot of other activities are given up, and if someone looks after your domestic needs – shopping, preparing meals, cleaning and laundry. For some people, getting back to some sort of work, even if part-time, will have positive results in terms of their mental well-being and will remove the threat of isolation, feelings of uselessness and invalidism. A return to part-time work may end up paying for home help, child care, etc., leaving no money to spare but offering great psychological benefits because you are able to return to the world. But if there is any doubt about your ability to return to work without having a relapse, think carefully.

I struggled for a few months, working only one morning a week to maintain a minimum income, and found that it took all week to get over the exhaustion caused by one day of light work. Once I decided to stop completely and make the commitment to getting better, some slow recovery started.

A lot will depend on whether you are self-employed and therefore your own boss, or, if employed, on the attitude and sympathy of your employer. You should also consider whether you can really be effective in your job if you are still unwell. It may be that clients, pupils, patients or colleagues suffer on those days when you are struggling and mentally under par, even though *you* may believe you are doing a tremendous job.

Do not be too proud to claim state benefits.
Do not think your presence at work is vital for the world to go round.
Remember there are thousands of other hard-working, conscientious and clever people just like you who have had to stop working because of illness; you are not unique.

See if there is a way of working part-time, with the flexibility to rest or go home if you feel ill. Access to a couch somewhere at work, to have a sleep mid-morning or midday, may enable you to stay in your job.

What if your work is unpaid, and is essential? I am of course referring to that underrated profession called 'housewife/mother'. The reasons for stopping work and resting apply to you as well, but the practicalities are difficult. If you cannot run your home, shop, or prepare meals, the Social Services Department may be able to arrange a home help, especially if you live alone or are a single parent. You may be entitled to a home help even if you are supported financially, if your husband or partner has a busy job and is out most of each day.

If you require help with dressing, washing, meals, etc., you can claim Attendance Allowance. And you can claim this even if there is no one looking after you.

Someone who stays at home to look after you and who therefore cannot go to work may be able to claim Invalid Care Allowance.

If you have young children, and have no one to take them each day while you rest, Social Services may be able to arrange a child-minder for a few hours a day.

You can be assessed by someone from Social Services who will visit you at home. When you are being assessed and questions are being asked, remember how you are at your *worst*, even if the visit takes place on one of your better days. Be quite definite about how much disability the illness is causing. It is no good saying 'Sometimes I can stand for long enough to wash up,' if this is the exception rather than the rule. The problem with M.E. is in convincing people that your energy evaporates very quickly and is insufficient to provide for the most basic needs of living. You must describe yourself as you are at your worst, and not minimize or be apologetic about your disability. This advice also applies if you apply for Invalidity Benefit or Severe Disablement Allowance, or see a doctor for assessment for Mobility Allowance.

Local support services (mainly Social Service) can arrange occupational therapy, home helps, home visits by chiropodists, home aids, etc. The Social Service Transport Section organizes the Orange Badge Disabled parking scheme.

The Citizens Advice Bureau can advise on these and other services, and if necessary will visit you at home.

Summary of Benefits, April 1991

Booklet FB2, *Which Benefit?* is a total guide to Social Security and NHS benefits. Another useful booklet is FB28, *Sick or Disabled?* – both are available from post offices and DSS offices, and contain lists of other leaflets that cover more specific services.

1. Employed, and have paid Class I National Insurance:
   Statutory Sick Pay – up to 28 weeks, minimum 4 days
   Invalidity Benefit – after 28 weeks
2. Employed or self-employed, and have paid National Insurance:
   Sickness Benefit – up to 28 weeks
   Invalidity Benefit – after 28 weeks
3. Unemployed, or have not paid enough National Insurance contributions:
   Income Support (used to be called 'Supplementary Benefit')
   Unemployment Benefit
4. Unable to work for over 28 weeks, and ineligible for Invalidity Benefit, not having paid enough N.I. contributions:
   Income support
   Severe Disablement Allowance – if at least 80 per cent disabled
   Mobility Allowance – if unable to walk
   Attendance Allowance – needing constant looking after
   Invalid Care Allowance – carer spending at least 35

hours a week looking after someone who gets Attendance Allowance

(*Note* – the last three benefits listed above are going to change in April 1992 – see below.)

Mobility Allowance

To be eligible for this you must be unable or virtually unable to walk, or have a condition in which walking seriously harms your health – e.g. heart disease or severe M.E. It is not means tested, and is independent of other sources of income. Your local DSS office will send you the application form. You will normally be examined by a doctor who is not your own GP. It takes about two months to come through, if your application is accepted. It is paid to help a disabled person run a car, or take taxis, i.e. to be mobile. If your initial application is not successful, but you are seriously limited in walking ability, you can appeal, and it is a good idea to get your case backed by a letter from a consultant who has diagnosed you and has seen you recently.

Income Support

This is made up of the following:

personal allowance
plus disability premium, if ill over 28 weeks
plus premium payment (for people with special expenses)
plus possible housing costs payment

The Social Fund helps with exceptional expenses.

Help with NHS charges is available for those on Income Support or a low income: Free prescriptions, free dental treatment, sight testing, and help towards the cost of glasses.

Changes in Benefits

In April 1992 there are to be major changes to benefits for the disabled. At the time of writing full details are not available, but here is a brief outline:

1. Disability Living Allowance

   This will replace Attendance Allowance and Mobility Allowance for people under 65. It will be made up of two components which are not linked to each other, so you may qualify for either or both:

   The care component will be paid at one of three rates, and replaces the present Attendance Allowance. The new lowest rate will be paid to those who need attention for 'a significant portion of the day' (instead of all day) and to those unable to cook for themselves.

   The mobility component will be paid at one of two rates. The higher rate will need the same rules as the present Mobility Allowance, with the minimum period of award reduced to six months. The lower rate will be payable to those who can walk, but need supervision or help from another to walk outdoors.

2. Other benefits

   Disability Working Allowance will be a means tested benefit for those who are working.

   Attendance Allowance remains payable to the over-65s.

   Invalid Care Allowance will be payable to those caring for people receiving the higher and middle (but *not* the lowest) rates of the care component of the Disability Living Allowance.

Registering Disabled

The Register of Disabled Persons was set up by the Manpower Services Commission (MSC) to help disabled people to get employment. You can apply for registration whether you are in employment or not. Registration is voluntary, but some facilities are only available to those who are registered.

Applicants will be asked to produce medical evidence to support their application, or to have a medical assessment.

Registering as disabled with the MSC is not the same

as registering with the Social Services. You can get further information from your local Job Centre. Various benefits from registering disabled with the MSC can include adaptations to help with your work, help with public transport, easier parking, help with rehabilitation, and training schemes.

Mobility

You can apply for an Orange Badge disabled car sticker if you cannot walk more than 50 yards. There may be occasional days when you can walk over 50 yards without detriment, but if the disability is the rule rather than the exception, apply for the Badge. Application forms are supplied by the Social Service Transport Section, and will be posted to you in response to a phone call.

However, at the time of writing it is difficult to get Disabled parking concession (Orange Badge) unless you are getting Mobility Allowance. The problem for M.E. people is that most car parks are far more than 50 yards from essential places such as the bank or post office.

If you do qualify for a Disabled Badge, use it when you cannot walk; but if you luckily have a remission or some good days, do not abuse the Badge. The sight of someone parking on double yellow lines in busy traffic, with the Orange Badge displayed, then getting out and walking normally for a distance, enrages traffic wardens and other disabled people, and does our cause no good. I have found traffic wardens very helpful when I have difficulty parking and walking. It always pays to ask for help as politely as possible, and to explain your problem.

An Orange Badge can improve the quality of life enormously – visiting a bank, a hairdresser, the library, and friends whose houses abut yellow lines all become possible.

Two useful DSS leaflets are:

HB2, *Equipment and Services for Disabled People*

HB4, *Help with Mobility*

You do not have to go to a DSS office to find out what help you are entitled to. Phone your local Social Security Office and ask to be sent the relevant leaflets, or write to:

DSS
P.O. Box 21
Stanmore
Middlesex
HA7 1AY

The M.E. Association has produced two helpful booklets:

A Guide to Benefits

A Guide to Services and Resources – this describes the various services which exist in the community, outlines the main resources available to help M.E. sufferers, and suggests ways of maximizing the chances of getting help.

To obtain these, and information about their cost, write, with s.a.e., to the M.E. Association (address in Appendix A).

The *Disability Rights Handbook* has information on new allowances, the recently established Benefits Agency, and Poll Tax changes. It costs £4.50, and is available in bookshops.

Wheelchairs

You do not need to be totally unable to walk to consider getting a wheelchair. A wheelchair, plus someone to push it, can open up horizons for you if you cannot walk very far. You can potter round a shopping centre, visit art galleries, stately homes, or go for an outing in your neighbourhood. Trips away, holidays, all sorts of journeys may now be possible with a wheelchair. Apply to Social Services, or the Red Cross for the loan of one.

Caution – do not wheel the chair yourself.

M.E. affects the arms as well as the legs, and the wheelchair is meant to conserve your energy! The helper who pushes you will need a few practice sessions away from a busy road or pavement. A common mistake for the learner-pusher is to allow the chair to tip forward when going off a pavement, risking the occupant falling out. To negotiate pavements, steps, or bumps, the chair is tipped back so the weight is all on the main wheels. The other main rule in the wheelchair code is *brakes on when parking*. Your pusher needs to be reasonably fit, as well as willing – wheelchairs can be hard work, especially on uneven ground.

Many M.E. patients whose walking is quite limited shy away from the idea of a wheelchair, because they do not want to become, or be seen as, an invalid. Being an invalid is partly a state of mind and partly a way other people perceive you. Better to see the wheelchair as a useful tool to help you get out of the house and join in the rest of the world at times. When you have a remission or get better, you won't need it.

Walking Assistance

The best aid, other than a wheelchair, is a folding stool-stick which can be used as a walking aid and then unfolded easily into a seat when needed. It is absolutely invaluable if you get collapsing, aching legs when having to stand for any time. If you are halfway round a supermarket and feel dreadful and shaky, you can park yourself on the stool for a few minutes – also at the checkout, in queues in the bank, at bus stops, and railway stations.

This gadget is *not* the same as a 'shooting stick', which has a sharp point to go into the earth and a very small seat (devised to sit on while you watch others shoot game birds). These are quite unsuitable, as the sharp point will not stay put on a shop floor or pavement. The best stool stick is sturdy, with four non-slip rubberized feet and a strong canvas seat, and is made in different heights.

Stool sticks are obtainable from various retail outlets, including National Trust Centres, and some sports shops – those that supply things for hunting and shooting (the address of one supplier is given in Appendix A).

Travel

It is possible to go away on holiday with M.E., but obviously not while acutely ill. For some, a change to sea or mountain air, the sun, and new horizons may be enjoyable and benefit the health. For others, especially those who get vertigo and visual problems from movement, the journey may be too uncomfortable, and the need to adapt to new surroundings, a different bed and a new daily routine may be too much to cope with.

Air travel may seem quick and simple, but in practice it is the most stressful form of transport since the days of the bumpy stage-coach. If you decide to go for a holiday by air, it is wise to choose a time of year out of season, and to avoid those airports that are notorious for congestion or delays. It may actually be worth paying extra and travelling on a scheduled instead of a charter flight.

If you are unable to walk or to walk far – distances on foot at airport terminals may be ¼ mile or more – ask the travel agent, or the airline direct, to arrange a wheelchair or buggy. This will then be organized again at your destination airport. This needs to be arranged in advance, and confirmed a day or two before travelling.

In theory this all sounds fine, but beware of Gatwick Airport's newest, North terminal! Opened in 1988, modern, with arcades of dazzling shops and piped 'musack', this new terminal is a nightmare for the disabled, and indeed for anyone with a mountain of luggage and/or small children. Wheelchairs and luggage trolleys are not allowed on the inter-terminal connecting monorail train – they have to be left behind about 30 yards before entering the train. If you are lucky, someone different will meet you with another wheelchair at the other end. If you have a lot of luggage, tough. It is quite hard to find another trolley when you leave the monorail train.

Having researched this airport and its North terminal recently, going on a holiday to Greece, I heartily advise against using it unless you can contact the airport authorities in advance and find out if the rules have changed or if they have now arranged means for a disabled person to arrive at the plane without having to change wheelchairs and walk!

The other disadvantage of air travel, apart from the stress and noise, is the level of chemicals in aircraft and terminals. If you are chemically sensitive, then you may feel quite unwell for a day or two after the flight. Some sufferers are adversely affected by the drop in pressure in the aircraft (this may particularly affect those with breathing problems).

Side-effects of air travel, or indeed any travel where increased exposure to chemicals and stress occurs, can be helped by taking extra vitamin C (1–3 gm) before and during the journey, and by drinking plenty of water.

Travelling by train is probably better than by air, or coach, or car on long motorways. British Rail issue Disabled Persons Railcards, which provide a discount of 30 per cent on railway tickets for both the holder plus an escort. If you receive Mobility Allowance or Severe Disablement Allowance, you can apply. If notified in advance, BR staff will help you on the train and meet you with a wheelchair or 'buggy' at the other end, which whisks you through the crowds in comfort to a taxi or, if someone is meeting you, to a waiting car.

There is an informative leaflet, *British Rail and Disabled Travellers*, available from BR stations. If you do not drive, cannot afford to run a car, and do not have a carer or relative to drive you, then rail transport for long journeys is relatively painless, provided you ask BR for help at least a day in advance, and do not travel just before a bank holiday, or during school half-term!

When travelling, and if using assistance, do not try

and walk some of the way – the staff will not understand if you say you can walk a few yards but get tired. The type of disability produced by M.E. is very difficult for most people to understand, especially as we don't have crutches or callipers.

A problem encountered by some in long car or coach journeys is that of petrol or diesel fume pollution entering the vehicle; this is worst of all on busy roads or in traffic jams. A car with a filter at the air intake may help, but these are rare. It may help to be aware of this problem, and close all windows and vents when stuck in slow-moving traffic.

The decision on whether on not to travel, and how, is a very individual matter. But the opportunity to travel and escape from four walls should not be dismissed out of hand. A journey will need much more planning and thought than it did when you were well, but is still possible. I know of at least two M.E. sufferers, both hardly able to walk, who have had enjoyable trips abroad with the help of a wheelchair, other people, and schedules that still allowed plenty of rest.

House and Garden

There are lots of ways of making home life easier. Most energy-saving ideas come from fellow-sufferers, and in every copy of your local M.E. Society's newsletters you will find many helpful ideas. In the home, several obvious possibilities are:

If your bed is not on the same floor as the bathroom, have it moved there if you are in a bed-resting phase.

Do everything in the kitchen sitting down, if possible, by arranging a chair near a work surface for food preparation, and using a high stool at the sink for washing up, raising the washing-up bowl to the same height.

Collect everything in one container that you need for preparing a meal, e.g. washing-up bowl, or basket, and take them to the work area before sitting down.

Iron sitting down, or do not iron at all; there is very little that really needs ironing, or cannot be ironed by someone else.

If your finances allow, consider investing in a machine that chops and mixes food – a food-processor. Chopping vegetables can be exhausting, and the temptation would then be to live on toast and tinned food, which are not good for you.

If you are spending a lot of time in bed and are well enough to talk on the phone, get a phone extension (which you can switch off) by the bed. There are telephones aids for disabled people; a shoulder rest to save you holding up the receiver is very helpful. Have a very comfortable armchair in the bedroom by a window, ask someone to fix a bird table within view, and get some binoculars. Make your bedroom cheerful, warm, and homely to be in.

In the bathroom, have a stool or chair to sit on while drying after a bath or wash, or while undressing. If having a bath is too exhausting, a stool or chair under the shower is a solution. If there is no shower, try sitting on the stool in the bath, and have a bowl of warm water on a chair next to the bath. Scoop the water out with a large unbreakable container and slosh it over yourself, or ask your helper to do this for you. You can wash all over and rinse while sitting down, and feel fresh and clean afterwards. (In countries with limited water or no plumbing, this is the normal way to have a warm shower!)

Make sure the bathroom is warm for this all-over wash. This 'two chairs and a bowl' method is much less exhausting than a bath or standing by a basin. A non-slip bath mat is essential for any method, especially if you have problems with balance or co-ordination.

In the garden, have a very comfortable seat at hand, such as an adjustable sunbed, to lie or rest on. Doing gentle gardening can be very therapeutic to the soul if one is well enough, and it gets one out of the house into the fresh air and light, but there must be somewhere to rest at frequent intervals. There is a gardening stool for disabled people available, which one sits in and is still able to weed or use tools at ground level. A local garden supply centre should have details on such an aid. Even in a wheelchair, it is possible to work in raised beds and borders. Sowing and 'potting on' can be done in a greenhouse from a chair.

The main enemy action in the garden is bending over or crouching, which places great strain on your thigh and back muscles. Sitting on newspaper or other waterproof layers beside a section of plant bed is preferable.

Keeping Warm

Keeping warm is very important. In M.E. the circulation is usually bad, the body's thermostat doesn't work properly, and a lot of energy can be wasted in fighting the cold – energy that is needed for other vital functions. Nor is the problem confined to the winter, at least not in the UK, where temperatures can drop low enough to require heating, hot water bottles and electric blankets from June onwards throughout summer.

Remember to keep your feet warm at all times, and that 30 per cent of body heat is lost from the head. A woolly hat may be helpful, not only for outside, but in bed at night, or while indoors in cold weather. Several thin layers of clothes are always better insulation than a few thick ones, and extra layers should always be at hand to put on wherever you are, especially if away from the house. A sudden feeling of chilliness can strike at any time, regardless of the weather, often due to a drop in blood-sugar, or rapid exhaustion; your body temperature may bear no relation to whether you feel hot or cold! A sudden attack of iciness may mean you need to have something to eat, and to have a sleep.

Just because others in the household may be comfortable in shirtsleeves doesn't mean that it is warm enough for you. But rather than turning up the central heating (70°F/21°C is the maximum advisable), you should wear more clothes and pay attention to keeping your head, feet, and neck warm. It is still important to have some ventilation in the home, even in cold weather.

In cold weather it is sensible to have a stock pot of soup or a stew on the go. This supplies instant hot food with minimal time to be spent in a cold kitchen just before a meal. Certain foods have warming properties, such as ginger, cayenne pepper (caution – you only need a pinch), most curry spices, peppers, garlic, and brown lentils. These foods will warm you whether they are taken hot or not, and are good to include in stews or soups.

Heated mini-blankets, or heat pads, are a good way to supply warmth to the back, chest or tummy as needed if you are cold and have stiff or painful muscles. An electric blanket is marvellous for providing instant warmth when you get into bed, all the year round. Do make sure it is safe, though, and do not leave it switched on if it is an underblanket.

A warm bath or shower is good for warming, also for improving circulation and lymph-fluid flow and for removing waste products that the body gets rid of through the skin via the sweat. Many people forget that the skin is an organ that eliminates toxins and body waste, so sweating a lot when you are ill is not a bad thing. The kidneys, skin, colon and lungs all get rid of waste, plus water, which needs to be replaced in ample amounts.

However, a hot bath (over 99°F/37°C) is *not* recommended if you are ill, weak, or have any heart symptoms, because of the extra strain the excessive heat puts on the circulation. Unless specifically advised as part of hydrotherapy treatment, bath water should not be hotter than body temperature.

Part of the benefit of a bath or shower comes from a rub down all over when drying: this stimulates circulation of lymph, the fluid carrying the white cells. Drying yourself may be the most exhausting part of the washing process, and you may need to ask for help with this if there is much muscle pain and fatigue. It's better to forget modesty and have some help, rather than forego a regular bathe which does much good to morale and body.

Many additional helpful hints will come from other M.E. people whom you meet or telephone through local groups. As someone said, necessity is the mother of invention! Only someone with the same problem as you can really advise you on how to solve it.

Chapter 20

Children and M.E.

Children and teenagers can and do develop M.E. Children around the age of puberty seem most vulnerable (it is rarely found in children under the age of 5). Males and females are equally affected. The most serious effect is the cognitive dysfunction, which causes loss of education at a critical age. Even if the child is well enough to attend school, his or her performance in class and at exams falls behind.

The most common, and serious, misdiagnosis is 'school phobia'. A physician who has made a particular study of childhood M.E. is Dr David S. Bell, a paediatrician at Lyndonville, NY, USA, where there was an M.E. outbreak in 1985: '104 patients were identified who retrospectively met criteria (for CFS). 44 patients were in the 6–7 year age group. All were followed up for at least two years, when only four children had made a complete recovery.'

Children can also suffer from having a parent or sibling with M.E. They may feel left out, neglected, or unloved if more attention is given to a sick brother or sister, or if an ill parent has not the energy for good parenting. A child may suffer anguish at seeing a parent devastated by M.E., and may demonstrate this by bad behaviour, depression or sleep disturbance. It is important to remember the silent suffering of a young child where another member of the family has severe M.E., or any other chronic illness.

The onset of M.E. in a young person does not differ from that in an adult, although it is usually more acute, and follows an infection which is frequently present among school classmates. Dr Bell has observed two patterns of onset: those aged 5–12 tend to have a gradual onset, and adolescents are usually acute in onset following a flu-like illness. This makes diagnosis much more difficult in the younger age group. M.E. in children may be misdiagnosed as: migraine, abdominal pain syndrome, atypical epilepsy ('petit mal'-type seizures are more common in childhood M.E. than in adults), juvenile rheumatoid arthritis, and school phobia.

The clinical features and chief symptoms are no different from those experienced by an adult, although some of the nervous system symptoms may not be so obvious because a child is less likely to complain specifically of poor memory, poor concentration, or depression. These symptoms manifest instead as poor school performance.

Children tend to become ill rapidly if they develop an infection, and they will tend to have a higher temperature than would adults, and more severe symptoms. They react more rapidly than adults, but also recover more quickly from most acute infections. So it is noticeable when a youngster who has been laid low with a feverish illness fails to make the expected recovery in a week or two.

Problems of Children with M.E.

Diagnosis

The agreed criteria for diagnosing M.E./CFS include a length of illness of six months or more. Clearly, parents want to know what is wrong before their child has been ill for six months. Bearing in mind that physical activity makes the condition worse, and that rest early on may allow early recovery, it is obviously very important to get an assessment and provisional diagnosis when the child is not recovering as expected from an infection – this may be a diagnosis of a 'Post-viral Fatigue Syndrome'

(PVFS), made on the basis of the child's history and the absence of signs or positive test results for any other disease.

Once this diagnosis has been reached, maybe as early as six or eight weeks after the onset of illness, the child can be allowed to rest as needed, the school is informed, and pressure to go to school or do sports is removed. The diagnosis may become M.E. if the illness continues for many months, with classical symptoms of muscle fatigue and brain disturbance.

Some GPs and school doctors are still reluctant to diagnose PVFS, or M.E. or CFS in a child. They may either still consider that M.E. is psychological, or believe that it is a condition mainly experienced by the over-twenties.

Although M.E. itself is less common under age 20, many children suffer prolonged fatigue after an infection; some of these do continue to be unwell, or even deteriorate, and have the classic M.E. syndrome for a year or more. It is tragic for a child and his or her parents to have to battle with doctors and education authorities for months, while the child may try to attend school and live a normal life but keeps on relapsing and possibly deteriorates.

If your doctor is ignorant about M.E. and other post-viral syndromes, or is simply unhelpful, you can do several things:

a) Contact one of the national M.E. support groups (addresses in Appendix A), and obtain information for the doctor about the illness.
b) Change to another doctor.
c) Find out if there is a specialist in your area who understands M.E., and ask for a referral, or arrange for a private consultation.

Because there are often strange psychological symptoms, and the fatigue leads to inability or reluctance to go to school or to do homework, some doctors and education authorities find it easier to diagnose 'school phobia' rather than suspect post-viral fatigue syndrome. They may also try to diagnose some family-behaviour problem to explain the child's change in behaviour.

Factors which help in the diagnosis of PVFS/M.E. are:

- a child who was enjoying school and sports has changed since becoming ill – the psychological problems are new and out of character
- the association of what was obviously an acute infection – in the child, or in the family – with the onset of the illness. The infection may have given few symptoms in the child, but others in the family may have had it more severely
- worsening of the child's symptoms after exercise or after mental exertions – e.g. after sports or an exam
- fluctuating symptoms from week to week or day by day
- aches and pains quite unlike anything the child has had before
- symptoms not improved by going on holiday, or at weekends; in other words, normal family life and exercise out of school are just as bad as school activities. A child with school phobia would be expected to make a dramatic improvement during holidays.

Before the consultation with a GP or specialist, write down the history of the onset of the illness, and any of the above factors if they apply to your child.

Do not be fobbed off by a doctor if you think your child has PVFS/M.E. Insist that adequate tests are done to exclude other physical illnesses, and if there is no diagnosis, ask what is making your child ill.

If the doctor does not know about M.E., and finds no physical signs of illness, and blood tests are normal, the next stage may well be a referral to a child psychologist or psychiatrist. This assessment will be quite exhausting for the child. However, many parents do agree to such an assessment; a properly-trained and skilled psychologist should be able to diagnose that the child has an illness rather than a purely psychological upset. The results of such an assessment may actually strengthen your case.

Management of Children with PVFS and M.E.

Complete physical and mental rest must be encouraged at first. For the first few weeks or months, general nursing care, as would be done for any ill child, is appropriate. The appetite may be poor, there may be nausea, constipation, diarrhoea, tummy pains, or severe headache. Do not use aspirin for pain, rather a small dose of paracetamol, or homoeopathic remedies if your doctor uses them. Constipation seems to make symptoms worse, possibly due to toxins absorbed from the bowel, so encourage plenty of fluids, and as much vegetable and fruit intake as possible – a liquidizer for making vegetable soups is invaluable.

Try and avoid sugar, 'junk food', Coke, and other non-nutritious things favoured by children. The diet guidelines of Chapter 11 apply to children, and adequate protein intake is especially important for weight to be maintained and growth to continue.

Problems arise when the child appears to make some recovery, and wants to do activities with friends, or to go to school and behave normally. You cannot force the child to stay in bed or in the house all the time; yet you cannot stand back and watch uncontrolled behaviour which will inevitably lead to a relapse.

The child's friends may be unsympathetic or even cruel when they see their pal going to school for half a morning, looking quite normal, then having to go home to rest for the remainder of the day. Keeping up with the peer group is very important for children and teenagers, and the loss of friends and activities shared with them can be as damaging psychologically as the pain and other symptoms.

When the child is getting better enough to want to go and do things, then a diary is a good idea, so that he or she can learn for him- or herself what the limits of the illness are at the time.

A frank discussion about the illness, what has caused it, how it affects the body and mind, and the likelihood of getting better, is a good idea at this stage. This will also dispel fears about other diseases such as cancer or heart disease or leukaemia, which may be preying on a young mind. With many TV programmes about illness, youngsters may know a lot about serious disease at an early age.

A plan of rest and activity for the child can be discussed among the whole family, so that he or she is involved to some extent with managing the illness. Brothers and sisters, and friends, should be encouraged to include the child in any discussion of what is going on in school and in their activities.

School, Education

Hopefully, once you have a diagnosis the school authorities will be understanding and co-operative about any restricted ability to attend school. There is a need for flexibility, and in some cases a compromise is needed so that part-time attendance is possible.

Avoiding sports such as gymnastics, team games and athletics is mandatory until it is clear that improvement is virtually permanent. As with adults, children and students who have M.E. will find that the less physical activity undertaken the more energy will be available for the brain. Some mental functioning may be possible so long as there is little physical exercise.

In theory, a home tutor should be a useful solution for children who are well enough to do some learning but cannot cope with the stress and noise of a full classroom. In practice, home tutors are rather scarce, and may not be easy to arrange. Sometimes a parent may be able to supervise some work at home provided by the school, done at a pace the child can manage.

Thanks to the work of the M.E. Association, Education Directors and their Special Needs Advisors have all been sent information about M.E. Information also been sent to the Association of Clinical Psychologists and to the Advisory Centre for Education (ACE) in the UK.

The Advisory Centre for Education (address in Appendix A) is a national independent education advice service for parents of children at state schools. They can give advice about legal rights, the roles and powers of Local Education Authorities, and where necessary provide support for legal actions.

In some areas, there may be enough M.E.-affected families to get together so that affected children and adolescents can meet or receive home tuition together.

It is enormously helpful for an affected youngster to have friends who have the same problems, even if the communication is by post. As with adults with M.E., the knowledge that there are others like you relieves the isolation.

At the moment, no one has come up with any magic cure for young people with M.E. The basic principles of management are no different to those that are advised for adults. Nutritional supplements are beneficial, at a dosage about half those suggested for adults. Multivitamin and mineral preparations for children are available, in chewable or liquid form, at most chemists and health food shops.

The disruption to schooling and social development which results from getting this illness as a child or adolescent is serious. At an age when things move on quickly, to have to drop out of life for a year or more can have long-lasting consequences. The pressures on youngsters to succeed – at sports, with classwork, in national exams and at university are great, reflecting the intense competition for jobs that awaits school-leavers and university graduates.

Perhaps it is not only the viruses that are causing M.E.

in children. Perhaps, in those worst affected, the tragedy resulting from the disease is yet another by-product of a society that places so much emphasis on achievement and material success; a society in which the opportunities to attain these things are restricted by high unemployment, and the demand for paper qualifications for virtually every job.

The M.E. Association (UK) now has a working party looking into all aspects of M.E. in young people under 25. They would like to hear from young M.E. patients or their carers, and are concerned about the needs of severely affected cases (address in Appendix A).

The following is a tragic case history, which will hopefully have a happy ending. Few children are as badly affected as this one, but young children can develop M.E. and remain ill for some years.

Ean's Story (told by his mother)

'May, 1986 – Ean fell ill after returning from a school trip; he was then 11 years old. His father and I both developed the same bug – swollen glands and nausea. Then in August we were on holiday by the sea. Ean was very sick and had diarrhoea for 24 hours, and was in bed for several days, as he began to feel achy and so tired. A trip to the zoo was a disaster, as the walk up the drive from the car park was just too much, he was exhausted and in tears with tiredness. He *never ever* got back to his real self; however he did start his new school and seemed to settle in well.

'15th Sept. – He was ill at school, burning up, headache, sore tummy, and his glands were still swollen. Teachers and other pupils were all ill with the same thing. Ean did not improve, he had bad headaches, sore throats, felt sick all the time, and sweated very heavily. He had very acidy-smelling breath, especially in the mornings, and poor appetite because of the nausea. Tests for glandular fever were negative. Later blood samples showed there had been a huge virus infection.

'13th Nov. – We saw Dr B. (a paediatrician) for the first time at the hospital. Ean had been ill now for six months. He had a brain scan, which was normal, and more blood tests.

'Christmas, 1986 – He began to lose his balance and started to drag his right leg. His legs seemed to be getting very weak, he still had nausea, and could not sleep.

'7th Feb., 1987 – Ean was no better, and his legs were weaker. As we live on the Isle of Man, we flew to Liverpool, where he'd been referred for a second opinion. We had a wheelchair and lift on and off the plane. He was examined and had blood tests, X-rays, brain scan, EEG, etc. These were all clear, and when we saw the specialist, he said Ean had Post-viral Fatigue Syndrome, and although this could be worse than the actual virus, he felt sure Ean would make a good recovery.

'Back home Ean was prescribed Optimax, (which we found out was for depression, and was not recommended for children), also Motillium for nausea, but he had so many side effects from these two drugs that we stopped them.

'April – Ean had all the same symptoms, but was getting worse. The paediatrician suggested we see a psychiatrist, to help keep his spirits up. Ean has never been depressed.

'Our G.P. suggested some very gentle leg exercises to try and keep the muscles going for when he started to feel better. We only went to physiotherapy once, as he found it so exhausting. We carried on with some of the exercises at home, but it made him feel more sick, tired and sore, and the bad breath came back.

'May – We took Ean to see Dr C. (a psychiatrist). He said that the virus which had affected Ean could be Coxsackie B, as this can cause disability like polio, but that you do get better from it. He also said that only complete and utter rest could cure it, and that this could take up to two years.

'July – We flew to Liverpool again for tests to be repeated. No tests were carried out, only an examination, and one of the staff told Ean there was "nothing wrong" with him and he would be walking in two weeks. The Liverpool consultant felt it was a psychiatric problem, and that Ean would be better in a psychiatric ward, removed from the environment in which he had become ill. However we did not accept the psychiatric treatment offered, and took him home.

'Back at home Ean was admitted to our local hospital to have the tests we had expected in Liverpool. The admission turned into a three-week Hell. The only test carried out was a lumbar puncture, the result of which was normal.

'They started giving him physiotherapy, which made him feel really ill, the pain brought tears to his eyes, but he was told "not to be a baby". Ean couldn't grip a spoon or fork any more, and could hardly lift his arms. He was forced to feed himself – this would take him ages, and his food would go cold. His voice was now getting weaker and it was often too tiring for him to repeat something. He would tell us he couldn't put up with much more. No one else but us believed how ill he really felt.

'Soon after this, we were given an article from a magazine called "What is this scourge called M.E.?" There in black and white were all the symptoms our son had – mental confusion, headaches, sore throats, sickness, vivid dreams, heightened sensitivity to light and sound. Here at last was the answer; we now felt we had found out what was wrong.

'12th Aug. – We went to see Dr Morgan-Hughes at the National Hospital for Nervous Diseases, London, where after an hour's consultation and an examination he said Ean was a severe case of M.E. or Post-viral Fatigue Syndrome. We were pleased to have a diagnosis. Dr Morgan-Hughes said it could be years before Ean was really better, that school was out for the foreseeable future, and that physiotherapy was wrong until he started to show an improvement; he said he would write this in his letters to the doctors at home.

'End of Sept. – Ean needed to have laxatives every fourth night. He also started to cough when he came into contact with smoke, or car fumes, especially diesel from buses and lorries if they passed us on our walks in his wheelchair. Grass-cuttings, perfumes and washing powders would all make him sneeze, and set his body shaking as though his balance had gone. His voice became so weak that it was just too exhausting for him to repeat anything. His fingers were now curled into a fist, and it was too painful to ease them out. We knew that the psychiatrist was trying to get a response to his questions that would show that it was something in Ean's mind that was making him ill. We have always believed, and still do, that our son is physically ill, it is not in his mind, and we will go on and on fighting for him.

'October – Ean had huge ulcers on his lips. He got confused if too many questions were asked at once, TV and flashing lights hurt his eyes, he had to wear dark glasses. One day the psychiatrist called, and amazed us by saying he still didn't believe Ean had M.E.

'We decided to take Ean privately to see Dr Morgan-Hughes again in London, as since August Ean's voice had gone altogether, and he could no longer open his fingers.

'21st March, 1988 – We went to the National Hospital for Nervous Diseases in London again. Blood tests, brain scans, X-rays, EEG were carried out, and all were fine. All the doctors there said he had a physical illness, and always said he had M.E.

'We were asked to speak to a psychiatrist, a Dr Wellesley, who was doing research on people with M.E. He never even saw Ean – after hearing the history of Ean's illness, he told us "Children do not get M.E." We disagreed with him, but he asked a top child specialist at Great Ormond Street Hospital to come (Dr Wellesley had still not seen or examined our son).

'Next day the child specialist, a Dr L., came; he also did not examine Ean. After listening to our story of how Ean's illness had progressed over the past 18 months, he said that he saw 12 children a year like him. We thought that he meant children with M.E., but later had our doubts. He suggested a combination of medical and psychiatric treatment, so Ean was admitted to the metabolic ward in Great Ormond Street hospital to start speech therapy and physiotherapy.

'Another psychiatrist told us that the whole family needed to attend for "family therapy" sessions. I explained this would be impossible because of the cost and distance from home. The doctor wouldn't accept this, and kept telling me that without these family sessions Ean would never get better, and that we would not be able to cope with him getting better! I said that if we as a family could cope with our son becoming ill, I could assure him we could cope with his getting better.

'Ean started treatment. The speech therapist would sit him in front of a computer for an hour. The bright green screen and the concentration needed would give him a bad headache. He then had to go for physiotherapy for over an hour, forced to stand for the whole time. He was shattered and ill afterwards.

'We went to see the ward the psychiatrist wanted to put Ean in. The door had a combination lock on it, children sat in a classroom glassy-eyed, and one girl was literally ripping her room apart, cowering in a corner, screaming. It scared all of us, and having seen the ward we could only consider Ean being admitted if the following could be agreed to in writing: No drugs without our consent, unlimited visiting by parents, use of M.E. diet and vitamins. The doctor could not agree to this, and said that we could take Ean back home, and arrange for him to have mild physiotherapy, speech therapy and counselling at home. But – in the letter to our GP, he wrote that we had ''discharged [ourselves]'', and ''kept denying Ean treatment''.

'May – Back home, we took Ean to see Dr Pickering, a well-respected homoeopathic doctor. After a long consultation he confirmed Ean still had M.E. and maybe some Candida infection. He gave us a diet to try, prescribed nystatin, vitamins and minerals, and asked to see Ean again in one month's time. We came away feeling we were at last getting somewhere, but how mistaken we were . . .

'Monday, 23rd May, 1988 – Our world came to an end . . . two social workers arrived on our doorstep, and *took Ean from us* under a ''Place of safety order'' – no warning, nothing . . . We weren't allowed to go in the ambulance with him, and did not even know when we would ever see him again. The order had been signed the day before (by a magistrate), and Ean was to be under the joint care of the island's psychiatrist and paediatrician.

'We were not allowed to see him for five days. Even now we still only have half an hour a day. When Ean was taken from us, even our parish priest was not allowed to see him. He was later allowed in to see Ean; he was our only link till we were able to see Ean ourselves. Ean was alone in a ward, could not move at all, could not speak, and yet had no way of getting help if he needed it. He had been told he had been taken from us because he was dying, and he sat waiting to see us with all that bottled up inside him.

'One day a doctor told him: ''There is nothing wrong with you, if you don't talk next week, you will be better off in our Mental Home, and never go home again.'' Ean was so scared he wet himself as he sat in his wheelchair, which he had never done since becoming ill. They still maintained that he did not have M.E., and said that they were just trying to scare him into talking and walking. One night we found him very upset – he had wet himself, as no one had asked him if he needed the toilet; he did not have a call button.

'Friday is the day he always dreads as he goes to the remedial pool; one day they let him go, certain he would put his arms out to save himself; he couldn't, so he went right under the water. The terror that child felt must have been indescribable. We have tried in vain to get the pool sessions stopped. He looks shattered each night on days he has had physiotherapy. His mouth is full of nasty ulcers again, his constant headaches are back, but no one ever asks him how he feels, so they never know. The nausea is much worse, and his eyes hurt because they removed his dark glasses. The noise of the other children hurts, due to his heightened sensitivity to noise.

'When he was in the National Hospital, London, they fitted his hands with splints, to open the fingers slowly, and you could straighten them and bend them for him easily. Now, with his splints off, his fingers are bending up again.

'Dr C., the psychiatrist, now says Ean has never had M.E. ''It's just school phobia, and an over-protective mother.'' We were told in London by Dr Wellesley, who never even saw Ean, that children do not get M.E. He is supposed to be an expert in the illness, too . . .

'Our latest hope in our battle to have our son returned to

us is the visit we have had by a paediatrician from Wales. He examined Ean, had a long talk with us, and said that Ean has had M.E., and still has it. Now we have to wait and see if the doctors here will at long last accept the diagnosis, or if we have to go and fight it out in court to get our son back home. We have the constant fear at the back of our minds that if we lose at the end of it all, he will be put in a locked psychiatric ward, which we know is the wrong place for someone so very ill with M.E.'

Mrs Proctor, August 1988

Postscript 1

On 20th October, 1988, after four months in hospital away from his parents, Ean was at last released back to his family. His condition was unchanged from May – if anything he was worse. A neurologist, Professor E. J. Field, had been allowed to examine Ean in September. His conclusion was that the child was a severe case of M.E. and that neither psychiatry nor hospitalization had any place in his treatment. Now Ean is receiving treatment again from a homoeopathic doctor, and his family wish to forget the nightmare and concentrate on helping him get better.

Postscript 2

May 16th, 1991 – I saw Ean today, not having seen him for 2½ years. What a good recovery he is making! He has recovered in almost every way, the one exception being his voice, which has not returned. A speech therapist said that his voice will probably return spontaneously, and an ear, nose and throat (ENT) examination found his vocal chords are normal.

Otherwise Ean can walk, run, swim, attend school full-time, has grown to 6 ft – he is now 16 – and has no symptoms of headache, nor food intolerances, nor mouth ulcers. He is cheerful, and has no psychological after-effects from his ordeal, thanks to the constant affection and support of his family, and the care of the homoeopathic physician who has treated him since his release from hospital. Ean's management included immunoglobulin intravenously (administered by Dr Lewis, the paediatrician from Wales who also diagnosed Ean's M.E.), then magnesium injections, an anti-Candida diet, vitamin and mineral supplements, nystatin, high doses of evening primrose oil, and a German herbal therapy called *Spargaryk*, which is still continuing. He also had gentle physiotherapy weekly until he could walk again.

The family have just won their long legal battle against the authorities who removed him from them when he was very ill. A select committee of Tynwald, the parliament of the Isle of Man, decided that the doctors and social workers involved had acted wrongly, and that Ean should receive compensation.

The outcome of Ean's story is happy, but has cost his parents years of anguish, because they were disbelieved and criticized as being over-protective and denying their son treatment. The verdict of the Tynwald committee will encourage many families who still live in dread of a 'dawn snatch' of their ill M.E. children by people with too much power and no knowledge or understanding (nor the will to learn) of this disease.

Chapter 21

Caring for Someone with M.E.

The illness of any member of a family inevitably adds to the strain on relationships within it. If someone has an acute illness, or an injury, or an operation, there is an expectation that he or she will get better after a predicted period of convalescence, and will return to more or less normal life. So the period of upheaval is seen as temporary, it has some sort of boundary; the illness or operation is usually definable and recognized, and the whole period of illness and recovery can often be coped with.

But if having M.E. is a sentence of unknown length, with no remission for good behaviour for the sufferer, it may be an equally long sentence for the people closest to the patient.

A lot of the difficulties with M.E. that result from adjusting to living at home, in one's community, rather than in hospital or in a nursing home, also apply to other chronic disabling conditions. The strain of caring for someone with heart disease, multiple sclerosis, a stroke, kidney disease, or cerebral palsy (there are many others) is no different from that of caring for a badly affected M.E. sufferer.

However, what makes the M.E. syndrome different is the *variability* and *unpredictability* of both the patient's physical state and mood. As a carer, one day you may rejoice to see the patient happily doing a little gardening, yet the next day may find you helping with dressing and washing. One day there are hours of sobbing and anguish, the next there is a calm person who does not realize what a dreadful day he or she gave you yesterday.

The unpredictability of M.E. makes planning for the future difficult. By the time the diagnosis is made, the patient has probably been unwell for six months or more. Can one confidently go ahead with plans that affect the household such as moving house, holidays, renovations, or job changes?

Fear of the future is always worse than the reality of today. There is probably a better chance of peace of mind if no long-term plans are made which cannot be unmade; living from day to day and letting the future take care of itself is to some extent a good philosophy for M.E. families.

In reading about relationships, the assumption may be that a man-woman relationship is referred to. I am, however, taking relationships to include those between friends, neighbours, and other relatives, as well as immediate family. By 'carer' I mean the person or persons most closely involved with providing practical and emotional support for the M.E. patient, be they spouse or neighbour.

In any close relationship there is a tendency for the emotional mood of one to have an effect on the other. If one person is sullen, withdrawn or depressed, the other thinks 'What have I done to cause an upset?' It is so natural to take the emotional moods of a loved one as a reflection of how he or she feels about us, and so very difficult to be a detached, though caring, observer.

So, if you are a carer, try and remember that your patient's rapid emotional changes are due to the illness, and not to changed feelings towards you or diminished need of you.

Because the life of the carer, as well as that of the sufferer, may be disrupted, this can lead to resentment on the part of the carer, and guilt for the sufferer. But both sides try desperately not to let these natural feelings show. Guilt at being 'such a burden' is common, and of course it just adds to all the mental suffering already experienced. The assurance of being loved and valued as a member of the household, in spite of being an apparently useless wreck, can reduce the guilt.

The resentment felt by a carer at having his or her own life disrupted by this interminable illness is a common emotion, and should not be underestimated. The carer then feels guilty about this resentment, cannot express it for fear of upsetting the patient, and so ends up irritable and moody. It is in this situation that a once open, loving relationship between carer and patient can deteriorate.

You as a carer may experience feelings of anger, resentment, frustration, or grief for many reasons:

because a loved one is ill and you don't know when he or she is going to get better,
because both your lives are turned upside down, and
because you may have to sacrifice your own job, time, hobbies or holidays in order to be able to care effectively.

These feelings are perfectly normal; you are not born to be a saint! What is wrong is to bottle everything up and do damage to yourself, the patient, and other members of the household.

The M.E. Association in the UK provides valuable support for sufferers through local groups, and a listening ear telephone service. But carers need support as well, and it may be helpful to talk to other carers, to people in the M.E. Association, or to anyone offering a sympathetic ear, if you feel you can't cope with the illness and the patient.

Sadly, a number of relationships do break down completely under the stresses created by M.E., leading to separation, divorce, loss of a lover or close friend, or children leaving home. I do not have the skills necessary to advise on how to prevent these separations; they happen to many people without M.E., but are harder to bear if a chronic illness is the main reason for the split.

Sometimes a relationship has been going wrong

anyway, before M.E. appeared, and in such cases a severance may *remove* a major stress, and later allow the patient a better chance of getting better. However, sometimes the human resources of loving and understanding develop in two people as a result of one of them getting M.E., and a lukewarm relationship may then grow into a much deeper and warmer one.

Possibly one of the most important aspects of some relationships to suffer is a sexual one. I do not think that a lessening of sexual desire is something confined to M.E., but may be a symptom present with many chronic illnesses. After all, becoming ill is a sign that the whole body-mind complex is not functioning properly.

A sick animal or child rests, following the body's need to conserve energy for healing. A sick adult human also stops expending energy on unnecessary activities. Sometimes there is not enough energy for digestion or for talking, so the body is certainly not going to give much priority to the act of lovemaking! In women who are ill, loss of interest in sex may be a protective mechanism (unconscious) against becoming pregnant while the body would be unable to cope with it.

The loss of sexual desire is a very common symptom with M.E., but is not something that people talk about readily to the family doctor. There are, of course, other ways of expressing affection as well as the sexual act itself. Some couples may succeed through compromise, such as finding occasions when the fatigue is not so great; using different techniques or positions; or perhaps by accepting that this one part of the relationship may have to be put aside for some time. Mutual understanding of why the problem arises, and accepting it as just another activity to forego for a while – just as one has to accept that long walks, late nights, socializing, etc. are activities to be postponed until the patient feels better – are ways of coping with this problem. (See also Chapter 18, page 255.)

It is enormously helpful for the M.E. patient if the

carer can demonstrate that he or she believes the patient has a genuine illness, and at the same time demonstrates the belief in possible recovery. It can be a bit difficult to draw the line between being supportive and helping in every aspect of living when needed, and in encouraging the patient to be an invalid.

There are times when the patient needs to be allowed to stretch his or her wings and try and do a bit more, and times when the carer needs to be firm and say 'That's enough, you must rest.' Balancing the functions of a protective nurse and a occupational therapist can be tricky even when looking after an illness which is predictable. With M.E., playing it just right is nearly impossible when your patient is so unpredictably up then down.

Here is some advice to the carer, given by someone with experience of this challenging job:

• The M.E. carer must have patience, compassion, resilience, and belief in M.E. as a mentally and physically crippling disease in varying degrees.
• You have to learn not to mind when people tell you you are being exploited by waiting hand and foot on someone who usually looks perfectly fit, e.g. in a wheelchair one week, and next week walking.
• You need to be aware of the varying limitations of the M.E. patient and be ready to step in, such as rescuing a patient from long and exhausting telephone conversations.
• Be prepared to help in all aspects of daily living, as required.
• If the M.E. patient, in desperation, behaves out of character, do not take it to heart, and learn not to be thrown by wide mood swings.
• Try to maintain the fine line between having a life of your own and yet still realizing the extent to which you are needed for moral as well as physical support.
• *In short – be a perfectly perfect person!*

Carers often feel isolated, and need help and support. Most people do not know exactly how the Health and Social Services work; if you or the person you look after need outside help, you may not know how to go about asking.

There are three sources of help to try first:

1. Your family doctor
   Do not neglect to tell your GP about your own health problems – a sick carer is entitled to medical help just as much as the patient. Ask about any help which may be needed with lifting, dressing, or bathing the person you care for.

   A district nurse may be asked to call and give advice.

2. The hospital
   If the M.E. sufferer is in hospital or attending an out-patients clinic, ask the specialist to explain any disabilities.

   Many M.E. patients prefer to avoid hospitals, though, as not all doctors and nursing staff understand what the illness is, and may want to institute physiotherapy. Hospitals on the whole are not good environments as regards getting plenty of sleep and avoiding chemicals!

3. Social Services
   The phone book gives the address and number of your local Social Services. You can ask:
   for a social worker to visit the home to find out what the patient's needs are,
   for information about what is needed, and
   what home help is available.

You may be entitled to financial help if you cannot work because of caring. DSS rules are going to change in 1992, however – see Chapter 19.

There are carers' groups in many areas – the M.E. Association may know of some, or else your local Social Services, Citizen's Advice Bureau, or local voluntary services may know of a group.

Useful addresses for carers are given in Appendix A. This last case history is of someone I have met. She and her family have shown great courage and patience for the 4½ years of her illness.

Clare's Story (told by her mother)

'In December 1986, Clare was a second-year university student, doing Psychology and English Literature. She lived in Halls of Residence, was generally fit, and enjoyed dancing and other active pursuits. On the morning of the 6th December she woke with what seemed to be flu. She returned to our house, spent eight days in bed, and felt exhausted. However, she seemed to recover, did her end-of-term exams, and felt reasonably well over Christmas.

'The flu returned on the 2nd of January '87 and, because she felt so exhausted, she went to the doctor on the 6th January. The GP took a blood test which showed a high antibody titre to Coxsackie B virus. Clare then returned to Halls, feeling decidedly more tired and much slower in her actions, some nights having to go to bed after tea. Another visit to the doctor and another blood test – this time there was no high Coxsackie antibody. In the meantime I had read about M.E. and asked if this was a possibility. The GP totally rejected this, told Clare she had a post-viral condition, that she should continue with her studies but not take any strenuous exercise (''Aerobics maybe, but squash no!'').

'During the period from February to the end of the second term, Clare's condition worsened, with only a few brief spells of remission. She had greatly slowed down, couldn't imagine walking very far, and was generally behind with her studies. During the Easter holidays she decided that she could no longer continue as a student, and notified the university authorities on 23rd April 1987.

'Around this time her GP referred her to a consultant at Ruchill Hospital who gave her a diagnosis of Post-viral Fatigue Syndrome or M.E. and estimated that it might take anything up to three years to get better.

'Gradually Clare ceased to be able to get up for meals. She

began to experience what she called ''a wobbly head'' – a frightening feeling where her brain seemed to be losing contact with her eyes. As well as the intense fatigue, other symptoms appeared in the following months – cold, almost wet feet, a sensitivity to light, with after-images, and sensitivity to sound combined with a ringing in the ears, culminating in a severe and constant headache in September.

'Any kind of stimulation seemed to produce pain for her. She was no longer able to tolerate visits from friends, and could have only limited contact with her family. Having a bath or washing her hair was beyond her. She suffered intense malaise and often felt that she was dying. From this time on her mobility disappeared, and she had to be pulled to the bathroom on a chair with rollers. Some days she was unable to sit up for meals and had to be fed.

'During this period Clare's father and I, in increasing desperation, sought help from various sources. A herbalist recommended an anti-Candida diet, which after five days made Clare feel very sick and caused vomiting. It also made her lose half a stone in weight, which, combined with the loss of muscle bulk, left her weight at 7 stone. She discontinued the diet as she felt unable to cope with the nausea and further weight-loss.

'In July a three-day stay in a homoeopathic hospital was equally unsuccessful. She returned home with a promise to the doctor-in-charge to continue on a wheat-free diet for some six weeks (which she did), and to try and sit on a chair for ten minutes per day, which she was unable to do. A physiotherapist was sent from the local hospital, but even sitting out on a chair for more than a few seconds caused Clare to break out in severe sweating, so this was discontinued.

'Autumn 1987 came round and Clare's symptoms were at their worst. She lay all day every day in a room with the curtains drawn and with wax plugs in her ears. An eczema-type rash developed on her face and was only kept at bay by daily applications of cortisone cream. The encephalitic symptoms were predominant – constant severe head pain, a sense of unreality, and nightmares. Another homoeopathic doctor, whose speciality was ''psionic medicine'', was contacted. In all telephone calls and letters he promised ''a significant return to health in the very near future''. After three months and no sign of recovery Clare's disillusionment was intense. Reflexology was equally futile.

'In January 1988 Clare was able to have the curtains opened – an hour a day initially, then throughout all the short winter days. She also decided to dispense with all diets, keeping her food balanced and additive-free (and cut out all chocolate, which she found had a bad effect on her). There had been no proof that the diets had helped her, and she felt her life was restricted enough. During March/April her headaches were as bad as ever, although her sensitivity to noise had abated somewhat.

'In April 1988 she heard that injections of Parentrovite were being tried with some success by an immunologist in Belfast. With the agreement of her GP Clare had six fortnightly injections which did seem to help her condition somewhat.

'She could now watch television for short periods, listen to the radio, have a bath and wash her hair once a week. She no longer needed her ear-plugs, and could cope with much more family input. The headaches and the ringing in her ears were still there, but were more intermittent and not so severe. This improvement was not dramatic, and was in fact imperceptible on a day-to-day basis.

'She then began taking amitriptyline, one of the tricyclics, to combat panic attacks (a *Horizon* TV programme suggested that it might be useful in some M.E. cases). Initially there were some side-effects, but these were outweighed by an overall improvement in her condition.

'However, after a year and a half in bed Clare was still unable to walk more than five steps, and her full recovery seemed a long way off.'

Postscript
'The following two years saw Clare make some progress, to being able to get up a little each day, being less sound- and

light-sensitive, and able to watch TV and speak on the phone. However her muscles were very weak and she was still mostly bedridden, and an increasing feature was anxiety/depression. A weekly visit from a psychotherapist seemed to do more harm than good. In October 1990 Clare agreed to accept treatment in the Psychological Medicine department of a local hospital. The doctor in charge took the view that M.E. is an organic illness, and was interested in alleviating symptoms.

'Clare stayed there five weeks, coming home two weekends. To begin with the staff didn't seem to do very much, and encouraged but didn't force any activity. They also changed her antidepressant to Clomiprimine. Despite the alien hospital conditions (patients smoking, lack of good sleep), we did notice a change in Clare over the time she was there. When she came home she began to try more things – going out in a wheelchair at first, then for short walks. She has gradually increased this activity and can go into town and for short trips in the car (she has given back the wheelchair). She still suffers from head pain and exhaustion, but nowhere near as severe or long-lasting as they once were. She also has big emotional troughs, and sometimes it seems harder for her to cope with the frustrations of being half well than it was when she was completely incapacitated. She hopes to return part-time to university in October of this year, but some days this seems unlikely

'I want to emphasize that she still has M.E., but maybe there was after four years some psychological element that had to be overcome before she could continue her progress to recovery.'

June 1991

Conclusion

In this book I have given an overview of the illness known once as epidemic neuromyesthenia and today as Myalgic Encephalomyelitis, Chronic Fatigue Syndrome, and other names I may not have heard of. It is still quite a mystery disease to most doctors; probably those most knowledgeable about M.E. are the sufferers themselves. There is more to learn about it every day, and it is important that M.E. people communicate with each other about things that help, and continue to support research and the education of non-believers. It is hard to believe this in 1991, but people afflicted by Multiple Sclerosis had to battle for years to have their illness accepted as being genuine. Many of them were regarded as malingerers or neurotics 20 or so years ago.

Perhaps one day there will be a 'treatment' for M.E., some medicine to take, some magic bullet to make it all better. Predictably, the main focus of current medical research into treatment is looking at ways of destroying the virus, or of regulating the confusion it causes the immune system. This is fine, so long as the basic principles of helping the self-healing process are also applied – rest, good food, fresh air and light, freedom from stress, and spiritual well-being.

In this book you will have noticed there is a word that is hardly used – that is the word *cure*. Perhaps you are disappointed, having hoped to find guidance to lead you to the magic remedy that will make you fit and full of energy to live the life you used to enjoy. Of course there are quite a number of M.E. people who get so much better that they consider themselves cured.

However, the possibility of relapse is always there, and it is really foolish for someone who seems to have recovered to push his or her body to the limits, or to go without sleep, or eat badly. The viruses that trigger off M.E. are still around, either having gone back to sleep (becoming latent) in your body, or still floating around in the community.

It is useful for anyone who has a chronic illness to consider the two terms 'health' and 'fitness', because they can be erroneously thought to be the same thing.

What is meant by being 'fit'? This is a state that is desired by athletes, and by people who want to be able to exert themselves without suffering ill effects. One's heart, lungs and muscles must be in perfect working order. Fitness is, however, a purely physical condition, and ignores the state of the mind and the soul. Someone can be apparently superbly fit for the task of running up mountains or having the endurance to run 25 miles, yet develop a prolonged illness following a viral infection. The most common cause of death among joggers seems to be heart attack.

Health, on the other hand, has a much more subtle meaning. I understand it to mean being integrated, balanced in oneself, at peace with the world, and content. A state of 'perfect health' – if it exists! – would mean the perfect functioning of body and mind, and a pure spirit. In M.E. the body does not function properly, certainly, but I do believe that there is more to health and life than a super-fit (or even half-fit) body.

I know two quite different people:

Mr Super-fit takes great care of his body; he runs or plays squash every day, and goes ski-ing or rock-climbing (both to top levels of endurance) at weekends and holidays. In his forties, he has the body of someone much younger. However, he is unhappy, tense, gets lots of headaches and vague symptoms, is antisocial, irritable and sometimes depressed.

Mr Laid-back is also in his forties. He is a bit

overweight, as he enjoys his food and wine. He loves his job of teaching young children, loves entertaining friends, is generous and always cheerful. Apart from walking and standing all day at school, and pottering in the garden, he takes no exercise whatsoever, and does not feel the need for it. He has not had a cold or a day off work for years, and has no bodily complaints.

Which of these men is healthiest? And which of them would cope best with getting M.E.?

As stated earlier on, health means 'wholeness'. The M.E.-stricken body may not be whole – sometimes it seems as though every part of it is broken down. But continually I am amazed at the wholeness of the spirit and personality of people I come across who are physically disabled in some way.

I can still recall vividly a patient I knew in a cancer and chemotherapy unit. She was only 38, her family were still young; she had an incurable cancer, was wasted and in a lot of pain. She had plenty to be resentful about, and to be scared of. Yet, following some sessions of healing with her parish priest, and knowing that many people were praying for her, she announced one day that she was healed. Her body did not miraculously rid itself of the cancer overnight; to a casual observer she still seemed desperately ill. What had changed was that she had accepted her condition, stopped being afraid, and felt completely at peace with her family, friends and her Maker. In her last few weeks of life she gave out so much love to those around her, that those of us caring for her felt enriched by her company. In one sense this lady *was* healed, and healthy.

So I think that one of the keys to getting on with M.E. is *acceptance* of how you are. This is not the same as wallowing in self-pity and saying, 'I'll never be any better.' No, it means saying:

M.E. has come into my life, it is a fact of life. I shall do what I can to improve the way I feel. I shall change my lifestyle, feed my body well, nourish my immune system, and give myself lots of tender loving care. I shall stop yearning for what I cannot have for the present, and count what blessings I have. If I listen to my body and look after myself I shall probably get quite a lot better in time. If I do not get back to how I used to be, I will nevertheless continue to be alive and able to appreciate many good things in life, by living from day to day and looking for joy in little things.

Those who cope best with M.E. seem to be the people who try to go along with it, who adapt to living with M.E., rather than fighting it. Ironically, there are other illnesses that one fights to get the better of – there is the saying 'fighting for life' against a severe infection or after an accident perhaps. But with M.E. one needs to be a bit less aggressive about the illness. There is a need for fortitude and resolution, certainly, and some discipline about not doing things. Because nobody who has M.E. ever knows exactly when he or she is going to get better, it is very important to be able to get on with some sort of life, even if it only 10 per cent of the amount of living there was before.

So, if it takes one week to complete a task, such as writing a letter, that used to take 20 minutes, never mind. The work done will have no less value!

Living with an illness such as M.E. is possible at all levels of affliction. Remember it does not kill, and that the majority do get somewhat better.

Whether or not you have any religious faith, you can appreciate that this prayer is one for M.E. people to learn and use:

God, grant me the serenity
to accept the things I cannot change,
Courage to change the things I can,
and the wisdom to know the difference.

Appendix A
Sources of Help

The M.E. Association

The M.E. Association was formed in 1976 by a small group of people with M.E. It has now grown into a large and professionally-organized charity, with local branches all over the UK.

The Association has three objectives – to find and offer support to people with M.E., to spread information about the illness, and to promote medical research. A newsletter, issued every quarter, gives up-to-date facts about current research, medical information, news nationally and from the local groups, and members' articles and letters.

The Association has helped fund several research projects in different medical specialities. It gives support of great value to people with M.E. through its central office and the activities of local groups. A confidential telephone help-line, Listening Ear, is manned by volunteer counsellors who are themselves M.E. sufferers.

The Association has actively campaigned for and achieved Government recognition of M.E. In order to promote greater understanding in primary health care, it has undertaken the circulation of diagnostic information to all GPs. Information packs have been sent to a wide range of professional and voluntary agencies with which sufferers may come into contact. These include Government departments, Directors of Education and Social Services, disability groups, Trades Unions, professional associations, and information services.

It also provides individual support for those seeking benefits and services. It has brought attention to those with special needs, such as children with M.E., and chronic severely affected patients.

The Association acts as a life-line for those who are isolated, despairing, confused and devastated by M.E. For many people with M.E., the first positive development comes when they find they are not alone, that they have got a real illness (even if this is not recognized by their doctor), that others have gone through similar experiences and are there to offer friendship, encouragement and hope.

The address to write to – with s.a.e., please – is:
M.E. Association.
Stanhope House,
High Street,
Stanford-le-Hope,
Essex SS17 0HA

M.E. Action

M.E. Action is a national membership organization offering help, information and other services to people with M.E. It also funds research, and campaigns to bring about the full recognition of M.E. as a genuine physical illness, as well as working for improved treatment, benefits and help for sufferers. The hallmark of M.E. Action is its acceptance of both orthodox and complementary medical approaches, its active campaigning and its treatment-orientated research programme. The membership is currently 4,200 (March 1992) and growing rapidly.

M.E. Action was founded in 1987 by Sue Finlay; its current President is Clare Francis, well-known yachtswoman and author. Since 1987 its main achievements include: the initial press and publicity campaign which caused M.E. to hit the headlines; the introduction of the first M.E. Patients' Bill in Parliament;

the creation of an M.E. journal – *Interaction*; a full range of member services; and the funding of the research into magnesium deficiency and M.E., and treatment by magnesium injections.

Members receive three copies per year of *Interaction*, which contains up-to-date medical and therapy information. Members also benefit from its telephone therapy help-line, postal libraries, legal service, and national network of local groups. Members are encouraged to participate in M.E. Action's campaigns and fundraising activities.

M.E. Action also produces a Therapy Information Pack which summarizes information about the various therapies that people with M.E. have found helpful. Other literature includes factsheets to give your doctor, employer and relatives, and an information pack for patients/practitioners about the magnesium treatment.

M.E. Action welcomes enquiries from patients and sufferers – as well as donations towards its work and research. Please send a large s.a.e. to the address below for a free factsheet about M.E. and membership details.
M.E. Action,
P.O. Box 1302,
Wells,
Somerset BA5 2WE
Tel. 0749 670799

Westcare

Westcare is a registered charity which provides information and services for people with M.E./PVFS and their relatives, friends, doctors and other health care professionals. It operates mainly in Bristol and the southwest, but no one is excluded. Its clinic in Bristol offers consultations with a doctor familiar with M.E., and with professional counsellors.

Westcare works co-operatively with other M.E. organizations and with the medical profession. Lectures and study-days are provided, and research is encouraged.

Westcare aims to develop further services, such as respite care. Anyone who may be able to help is invited to contact the Director.
Westcare,
15 Queen Victoria Road,
Redland,
Bristol BS6 7PE
Tel. 0272 738317

IFMEA

The International Federation of M.E. Associations (IFMEA) was founded by the Dutch and Norwegian patient organizations in August, 1989. Its main aims are to collect and disseminate medical information about M.E. and related disorders, to stimulate medical and scientific interest in M.E., and to further the activities of the national M.E./CFIDS Associations. Membership is open to all national patient groups; local organizations can join as Associate members. Membership is restricted to these national or local groups, however, and individual patient enquiries cannot be answered.
IFMEA,
23 Melbourne Road,
Twickenham TW11 9QX

Other Useful Addresses

M.E. Organizations World-wide
ANZMES Victoria,
P.O. Box 7,
Moonee Ponds,
Victoria 3039,
Australia

ANZMES N.S.W.,
P.O. Box 645,
Mona Vale,
New South Wales 2103,
Australia

M.E. Soc Inc,
S.A. Support Group,
Newsletter *Talking Point*,
P.O. Box 383,
Adelaide 5001,
South Australia

M.E. Vereniging,
Predikherenstraat 2,
3000 Leuven,
Belgium

Dutch M.E. Foundation,
Du Perron Straat 34 HS,
10 64 JT Amsterdam,
Netherlands

ANZMES (NZ) Inc.,
P.O. Box 35–429,
Browns Bay,
Auckland 10,
New Zealand
Produces *Meeting Place*, an excellent M.E. newsletter.

Norges M.E. Forening,
Eiksveien 96A,
1345 Osteras,
Norway

M.E. Association of South Africa,
P.O. Box 461,
Hillcrest 3650,
Natal,
R.S.A.

Stodgruppen,
Klinisk Ekologi,
Gothenburg,
Sweden

CFIDS (Chronic Fatigue and Immune Dysfunction
Society),
1401 East Seventh Street,
Charlotte,
N.C. 28204,
USA

Living with a Disability
ARMS (Action for Research into Multiple Sclerosis),
4a Chapel Hill,
Stanstead,
Essex CM24 8AG
Tel. 0279 815553

The Disability Alliance E.R.A.,
Universal House,
88–94 Wentworth Street,
London E1 7SA
Tel. 071–247 8776

Disabled Living Foundation,
380–384 Harrow Road,
London W9
Tel. 081–299 6111

MIND,
22 Harley Street,
London W1
Tel. 071–637 0741
Gives legal advice on rights of mentally ill patients.

Philips of Axminster,
Philips House,
West Street,
Axminster,
Devon EX13 5NX
Tel. 0297 32701
Supplier of stool-sticks

SPOD (Sexual Problems of Disabled People),
286 Camden Road,
London N7 0BJ
Tel. 071–607 8851

Nutrition

Biolab,
The Stone House,
9 Weymouth Street,
London W1N 3FF
Tel. 071–636 5959/5905
For an assessment of your nutritional status – doctor's
referral needed.

British Dental Society for Clinical Nutrition,
Glenrose,
Bernards Close,
Great Missendon,
Bucks
Tel. 02406 4601/5997
For information about testing for mercury sensitivity, etc.

Foresight,
The Old Vicarage,
Church Lane,
Witley,
Surrey GU8 5PN
Tel. 042 879 4500

Henry Doubleday Research Organisation,
Convent Lane,
Braintree, Essex
Advises on all aspects of organic gardening, and lists
suppliers of organic produce.

The Soil Association,
86 Colston Street,
Bristol,
Avon
Tel. 0272 290661

Women's Nutritional Advisory Service,
P.O. Box 268, Hove,
East Sussex BN3 1RW
Tel. 0273 771366
Can also offer advice on coping with PMS.

Dietary Supplements

Bach Flower Remedies Ltd,
Dr E. Bach Centre,
Mount Vernon,
Sotwell, Wallingford,
Oxon OX10 0PZ

Biocare Ltd,
54 Northfield Road,
Kings Norton,
Birmingham B30 1JH
Tel. 021–433 3727
Supplier of Mycopril (caprylic acid), an antifungal agent.

Lamberts Dietary Products Ltd,
1 Lamberts Road,
Tunbridge Wells,
Kent TN2 3EQ
Tel. 0892 46488
For orders from practitioners only; individuals should
write to the next address.

Nature's Best Health Products Ltd,
P.O. Box 1,
Tunbridge Wells,
Kent TN2 3EQ
Provides Lamberts' Supplements, which can be ordered directly by patients.
Many dietary supplements are also available in chemists and health food shops: the best are free of gluten, sugar, milk and additives – look at labels.

Renahall Ltd,
61 Lime Tree Avenue,
Rugby CV22 7QT
Tel. 0788 811454
Supplier of vitamin C powder.

Allergies
Action Against Allergy,
24–26 High Street,
Hampton Hill,
Middlesex TW12 1PD
Please send s.a.e.

Breakspeare Hospital for Allergy and Environmental Medicine,
High Street,
Abbot's Langley,
Herts

British Society of Allergy and Environmental Medicine,
34 Brighton Road,
Banstead,
Surrey SM17 1BS
Tel. 07373 61177

Alternative Medicine
British Homoeopathic Association,
27a Devonshire Street,
London W1N 1RJ
Doctors trained in homoeopathy.

National Federation of Spiritual Healers,
Old Manor Farm Studio,
Church Street,
Sunbury-on-Thames,
Middlesex TW16 6RG

Society of Homoeopaths,
2 Artizan Road,
Northampton NN1 4HV

Support
ACE (Advisory Centre for Education),
18 Victoria Park Square,
London E2 9PB
Tel. 071–354 8321

Samaritans,
17 Uxbridge Road,
Slough SL1 1SN
Tel. 0753 532713

Caring for the Chronically Sick or Disabled
Association of Crossroads Care,
Attendant Schemes Ltd,
10 Regent Place,
Rugby,
Warwicks CV21 2PN
Tel. 0788 573653

National Carers Association,
29 Chilworth Mews,
London, W2 3RG
Tel. 071–724 7776
Both of these are voluntary organizations offering support services for carers and their dependents.
Taking a Break – a guide for people caring at home (produced by King's Fund) – is available by writing to:
Taking a Break,
Newcastle upon Tyne X NE85 2AQ

Appendix B
Information for Doctors:
Diagnosis and Investigations

Conditions to Be Excluded:
Differential Diagnosis of M.E.

Metabolic myopathies
Myesthenia gravis
Polymyalgia, fibromyalgia
Motor neurone disease, other neuropathies
Multiple sclerosis
Various psychiatric disorders – e.g. schizophrenia,
severe depression, pre-senile dementia.
Nutritional deficiencies – e.g. of B_1, B_{12}, folic acid,
iron.
Thyroid disorders
Diabetes
Other endocrine disorders
Systemic Lupus Erythematosis
Rheumatoid arthritis
Connective tissue disorders
Coeliac disease
Crohn's disease
Chronic active hepatitis
Chronic pancreatitis
Coronary artery disease (especially if chest symptoms
are severe)
Pleurisy, other lung conditions
Chronic infections – e.g. TB, infectious mononucl-
eosis, brucellosis, Lyme disease, HIV/AIDS.
Parasitic infections – e.g. Amoebic dysentery,
bilharzia, giardiasis.
Cancers

Investigations

General Investigations Suggested for Patients Suspected of Having M.E.

Serial weight measurements
Serial morning and evening temperature measurements
Complete blood count, and differential white blood cell count (WBC)
Serum electrolytes
Blood glucose, creatinine, calcium, and phosphate levels
Liver function tests
Plasma viscocity
Creatinine phosphokinase
Thyroid hormone tests
Autoantibodies profile

Serology

EB virus antibodies
Viral capsid antigen (VCA)
EB virus nuclear antigen (EBNA)
ASO and ADBA titres
Serology for HIV/AIDS, cytomegalovirus and toxoplasma
ELISA IgM to Coxsackie B virus
Hepatitis A and B, and (if history suggests), a test for Lyme disease (caused by Borrelia burgdoferi).

More Specialized Tests

Tensilon test (for myesthenia gravis)
Muscle enzymes
Electrocardiograph, chest X-ray
T lymphocyte subsets, and NK cell function
Electroencephalogram
Muscle biopsy
Electromyogram

Enterovirus protein (VP1 – available only by request to the Department of Virology, St Mary's Hospital, Paddington, London).

Bibliography

Books

Crook, W. G., *The Yeast Connection* (Future Health, 1984).

Davies, S. and Stewart, A., *Nutritional Medicine* (Pan, 1987).

Gibran, K., *The Prophet* (Heinemann, 1926).

Howard, J. M. H., 'Muscle action, trace elements and related nutrients; the Myothermogram', in G. Chazot et al. (eds.), *Current Trends in Trace Element Research*, 1989, pp. 79–85.

Hyde, B., and Bergman, S., 'Chronic aspects of Akureyri disease', in *Post-viral Fatigue Syndrome* (Wiley, 1991).

Ott, J. N., *Health and Light* (Pocket Books, 1976).

Pauling, L., *How To Live Longer and Feel Better* (W. H. Freeman and Co., 1986).

Peters, T. J. and Preedy, P. R., 'Pathological changes in skeletal muscle', in *Post-viral Fatigue Syndrome* (Wiley, 1991).

Ramsay, A., *Postviral Fatigue Syndrome* (Gower Medical Publishing, 1986).

Periodicals

Acheson, E. D. (1959). 'The clinical syndrome variously called Benign Myalgic Encephalomyelitis, Iceland disease, and Epidemic Neuromyesthenia', *American Journal of Medicine*, **26**, 569–95.

Archard, L. C., Behan, P. O., Bell, E. J., Bowles, N. E., Doyle, N. (1988). 'Post viral fatigue syndrome: persistence of enterovirus RNA in muscle and elevated creatine kinase', *Journal of the Royal Society of Medicine*, **81**, 326–9.

Arnold, D. L., Bore, P. J., Radda, A. K., Styles, P., Taylor, D. J. (1984). 'Excessive intracellular acidosis of skeletal muscle on exercise in a patient with a post-viral exhaustion/fatigue syndrome', *Lancet*, **1**, 1367–9.

Arnold, D. L., Bore P., Radda, A. K. et al. (1985). 'Enhanced intramuscular acidosis during exercise by patients with post viral exhaustion/fatigue syndrome', *Neurology (Cleveland)* **35 suppl 1**, 165.

Beard, G. M. (1969). 'Neurasthenia or nervous exhaustion', *Boston Med. Surg. Journal*, **3**, 217–20.

Behan, P. O., Behan, W. M. H., Bell, E. J. (1985). 'The postviral fatigue syndrome – an analysis of the findings in 50 cases', *Journal of Infection* **10**, 211–22.

Behan, P. O. and Behan, W. M. H. (1988). 'Postviral fatigue syndrome', *Critical Reviews in Neurobiology*, **4**, 157–78.

Behan, P. O., Behan, W. M. H., and Horrobin, D. (1990). 'Effect of high doses of essential fatty acids on the postviral syndrome', *Acta Neurologica Scandinavica*, **82**, 209–16.

Behan, P. O., Goldberg, D. P., and Mowbray, J. F. (1991). 'Postviral Fatigue Syndrome', *British Medical Bulletin*, **47 no 4** 803–8.

Bell, E. J., McCartney, R. A., Riding, M. H. (1988). 'Coxsackie B virus and myalgic encephalomyelitis', *Journal of the Royal Society of Medicine*, **81**, 329–31.

Berrios, G. E., and Oemada, J. I. (1990). 'Depressive illness in multiple sclerosis: Clinical and theoretical aspects of the association', *British Journal of Psychiatry* **156**, 10–16.

Buchwald, D. and Komaroff, A. L. (1991). 'Review of laboratory findings for patients with chronic fatigue syndrome', *Reviews of Infectious Diseases*, **13 suppl 1**, S12.

Buchwald, D., Cheney, P. R., Komaroff, A. L. et al. (1992). 'A chronic illness characterised by fatigue, neurologic and immunologic disorders, and active human herpes virus type 6 infection', *Annals of Internal Medicine*, **116**, 103–113.

Butler, S., Chalder, T., Ron, M. and Wesseley, S. (1991). 'Cognitive behaviour therapy in chronic fatigue syndrome', *Journal of Neurology, Neurosurgery and Psychiatry*, **54**, 153–8.

Calder, B. D., Warnock, P. J., McCartney, R. A., Bell, E. J. (1987). 'Coxsackie B viruses and the post-viral syndrome: a prospective study in general practice', *Journal of the Royal College of General Practitioners*, **37**, 11–14.

Cavanaugh, S. V. A. (1984). 'Diagnosing depression in the hospitalised patient with chronic medical illness', *Journal of Clinical Psychiatry*, **45:3** (sec 2) 13–16.

Cheney, P. R. et al. (1989). 'Interleukin 2 and the Chronic Fatigue Syndrome', *Annals of Internal Medicine*, **110**, **4**, 321.

Cheney, P. R. (1990). 'Clinical findings in CFIDS-neurology', *CFIDS Chronicle*, **Fall 1990**, p. 8

Cheney, P. R. (1991). *CFIDS Chronicle Physician's Forum*, **1** no 1, p. 4.

Cox, I. M., Campbell, M. J. and Dowson, D. (1991). 'Red blood cell magnesium levels and the chronic fatigue syndrome (M.E.): a case-controlled study and randomised controlled trial', *Lancet*, **337**, 757–60.

Cunningham, L., Bowles, N. E., Lane, R. M. J., Dubovitz, V., and Archard, L. C. (1990). 'Persistence of enteroviral RNA in chronic fatigue syndrome is associated with the abnormal production of equal amounts of positive and negative strands of enteroviral RNA', *Journal of General Virology*, **71**, 1399–1402.

Daugherty, S.A., Henry, B.E., Peterson, D.L. et al. (1991). 'Chronic fatigue syndrome in Northern Nevada', *Reviews of Infectious Diseases*, **13 suppl 1**, S39–44.

David, A. S., Wesseley, S., and Pelosi, A. J. (1988). 'Postviral fatigue syndrome – time for a new approach', *British Medical Journal*, **296**, 696–8

DeFreitas, E., Hilliard, B., Cheney, P., Bell, D., et al. (1991). 'Retroviral sequences related to human T-lymphotropic virus type 2 in patients with chronic immune dysfunction syndrome,' *Proc. Natl. Acad. Sci.*, **88**, 2922–6.

Demitrack, M. A., Dale, J. K., Strauss, S. E. et al. (1991). 'Evidence for impaired activation of the hypothalamic-pituitary axis in patients with the chronic fatigue syndrome', *Journal of Clinical Endocrinology and Metabolism*, **73**, 1224–34.

Dowsett, E. G. (1990) 'M.E. escapes the myth of hysteria', *Hospital Doctor*, May 3, p. 23.

Dowsett, E. G., Ramsay, A. M., McCartney, R. A., and Bell, E. J. (1990). 'Myalgic Encephalomyelitis – a persistent enteroviral infection?', *Postgraduate Medical Journal*, **66**, 526–30.

Galland, L., Lee, M., et al. (1990). 'Giardia lamblia infection as a cause of chronic fatigue', *Journal of Nutritional Medicine*, **2**, 27–32.

Gow, J. W., Behan, W. M. H., Clements, G. B., Woodall, C., Riding, M., and Behan, P. O. (1991). 'Enteroviral sequences detected by polimerase chain reaction in muscle biopsies of patients with postviral fatigue syndrome', *British Medical Journal*, **302**, 692–6.

Grist, N. R. (1989). 'Myalgic encephalomyelitis; postviral fatigue and the heart', *British Medical Journal*, **11 Nov**, 1219.

Hickie, I., Lloyd, A., Wakefield, D., and Parker, G. (1990). 'The psychiatric status of patients with the chronic fatigue syndrome', *British Journal of Psychiatry*, **156**, 534–40.

Holmes, G. P. et al. (1988). 'Chronic fatigue syndrome: a working case definition', *Annals of Internal Medicine*, **108**, 387–9.

Ho-Yen, D. O., Carrington, D., and Armstrong, A. A. (1988). 'Myalgic encephalomyelitis and alpha-interferon', *Lancet*, **1**, 125.

Ho-Yen, D. O. (1990). 'Patient management of postviral fatigue syndrome', *British Journal of General Practice*, **Jan**, 37–9.

Hunter, J. O. (1991). 'Food allergy – or enterometabolic disorder?', *Lancet*, **338**, 495–6.

Hyde, B. (1989). 'Brain findings in M.E. patients', *The Nightingale*, 1 issue 2, 3.

Jamal, G. A., Hansen, S. (1985). 'Electrophysiological studies in the post-viral fatigue syndrome', *Journal of Neurology, Neurosurgery, and Psychiatry*, **48**, 691–4.

Jamal, G. A., Hansen, S. (1988). 'Post-viral fatigue syndrome', *British Medical Journal*, **296**, 1067–8.

Jamal, G. A., and Hansen, S. (1989). 'Post-viral fatigue syndrome: Evidence for underlying organic disturbance in the muscle fibre', *European Neurology*, **29**, 273–6.

Jenkins, M. (1989). 'Thoughts on the management of M.E.', *British Journal of Homoeopathy*, **78**, 6–14.

Jessop, C. (1990). 'Food and Environmental Factors in Disease', *Interaction* no. 6, winter 1990.

Josephs, S. F., Henry, B., Balachandran, N., et al. (1991). 'HHV-6 reactivation in chronic fatigue syndrome', *Lancet*, **337**, 1346.

Kajid, A. (1991). 'The effect of vitamin C on erythrocyte morphology', *Meeting Place*, **36**, 14–15.

Klimas, N. G., Salvato, F. R., Morgan, R., and Fletcher, M. A. (1990). 'Immunologic abnormalities in chronic fatigue syndrome', *Journal of Clinical Microbiology*, **28**, 1403–10.

Klimas, N. (1991). 'Elevated IL-1 levels found', *CFIDS Chronicle*, **Fall 1991**, 10.

Komaroff, A. L. and Buchwald, D. (1991). 'Symptoms and Signs of Chronic Fatigue Syndrome', *Reviews of Infectious Diseases*, **13 suppl 1**, S8–11.

Landay, A. L., Jessop, C., Lennette, E. T., and Levy, J. A. (1991). 'Chronic fatigue syndrome: clinical condition associated with immune activation', *Lancet*, **338**, 707–12.

Linde, A., Hammarström, L., and Smith, C. I. E. (1988). 'Ig G subclass deficiency and chronic fatigue syndrome', *Lancet*, 1, 885–6.

Lloyd, A., Wakefield, D., Boughton, C., and Dwyer, J. (1988). 'What is myalgic encephalomyelitis?', *Lancet*, 1, 1286.

Lloyd, A. R., Wakefield, D., Boughton, C. R., and Dwyer, J. M. (1989). 'Immunological abnormalities in chronic fatigue syndrome', *Medical Journal of Australia*, 151, 122–4.

Lloyd, A., Wakefield, D., Smith, L. (1989). 'Red blood cell morphology in chronic fatigue syndrome', *Lancet*, 2, 217.

Lloyd, A. R., Hickie, I., Boughton, C. R., Spencer, O., and Wakefield, D. (1990). 'Prevalence of chronic fatigue syndrome in an Australian population', *Medical Journal of Australia*, 153, 522–8.

Lloyd, A., Hickie, I., Wakefield, D., Boughton, C., and Dwyer, J. (1990). 'A double-blind, placebo-controlled trial of intravenous immunoglobulin therapy in patients with chronic fatigue syndrome', *American Journal of Medicine*, 89, 561–8.

Manu, P., Matthews, D. A. and Lane, T. J. (1991). 'Panic disorder among patients with chronic fatigue', *Southern Medical Journal*, 84, 541–6.

Matthews, R., Smith, D., Midgley, J. et al. (1988). 'Candida and Aids: Evidence for protective antibody', *Lancet*, 2, 263.

McEvedy, C. P., and Beard, A. W. (1970). 'Concept of benign myalgic encephalomyelitis', *British Medical Journal*, 1, 11–15.

Mena, I. (1991). 'Highlights of Los Angeles Conference', *CFIDS Chronicle*, **Fall 1991**, 30–1.

Montague, T., Marrie, T. J., Klassen, G. A., et al. (1989). 'Cardiac function at rest and with exercise in the chronic fatigue syndrome', *Chest*, 95, 779–84.

Mowbray, J. F., Yousef, G. E., Bell, E. J. et al. (1988), 'Chronic enterovirus infection in patients with postviral fatigue syndrome', *Lancet*, **1**, 146–9.

Mukherjee, T. M., Smith, K., Maros, K. (1987). 'Abnormal red blood cell morphology in myalgic encephalomyelitis', *Lancet*, **2**, 328–9.

Murdoch, J. C. (1987). 'Myalgic encephalomyelitis (M.E.) syndrome – an analysis of the clinical findings in 200 cases', *The New Zealand Family Physician*, **Autumn 1987**, 51–4.

Oldstone, M. B. A. (1989). 'Viral alteration of cell function', *Scientific American*, **Aug**, 34–40.

Pacey, P. J., Read, M., Peters, T. J., and Halliday, D. (1988). 'Post-absorptive whole body leucine kinetics and quadriceps muscle protein synthetic rate (MPSR) in the post-viral syndrome', *Clinical Science*, **75**, 36–7.

Perrins, D. J. D. (1990). 'The diagnosis of postviral syndrome', *Journal of the Royal Society of Medicine*, **83**, 413.

Peterson, P. K., Shepard, J., Macres, M. et al. (1990). 'A controlled trial of intravenous immunoglobulin G in chronic fatigue syndrome', *American Journal of Medicine*, **89**, 554–60.

Prasher, D., Smith, A., and Findlay, L. (1990). 'Sensory and cognitive event-related potentials in myalgic encephalomyelitis', *Journal of Neurology, Neurosurgery and Psychiatry*, **53**, 247–53.

Riley, M. S., O'Brien, C. J., McCluskey, D. R. et al. (1990). 'Aerobic work capacity in patients with chronic fatigue syndrome', *British Medical Journal*, **301**, 953–6.

Rosen, S. D., King, J. C., Wilkinson, J. B., and Nixon, P. G. F. (1990). 'Is chronic fatigue syndrome synonymous with effort syndrome?', *Journal of Royal Society of Medicine*, **83**, 761–4.

Schiffer, R. B. (1990). 'Depressive syndromes associated with diseases of the central nervous system', *Seminars in Neurology*, **10**, 239–46.

Simpson, L. (1989). 'Non-discocytic erythrocytes in Myalgic Encephalomyelitis', *New Zealand Medical Journal*, **102**, 126–7.

Simpson, L. (1990). 'Are M.E. and chronic fatigue syndrome the same disease?', *New Zealand Medical Journal*, **103**, 305.

Stenager, E., Knudson, L., and Jenson, K. (1990). 'Psychiatric and cognitive aspects of multiple sclerosis', *Seminars in Neurology*, **10**, 254–61.

Wakefield, D., Lloyd, A., Dwyer, J. (1988). 'Human herpes virus 6 and myalgic encephalomyelitis', *Lancet*, **2**, 1059.

Wakefield, D., Lloyd, A., and Brockman, A. (1990). 'Immunoglobulin subclass abnormalities in patients with chronic fatigue syndrome', *Paediatric Infectious Diseases Journal*, **9**, S50–3.

Wood, G. C., Bentall, R. P., Gopfert, M., and Edwards, R. H. T. (1991). 'A comparative psychiatric assessment of patients with chronic fatigue syndrome and muscle disease', *Psychological Medicine*, **21**, 619–28.

Wysenbeek, A. J., Shapira, Y., and Leibovic, L. (1991). 'Primary fibromyalgia and the chronic fatigue syndrome', *Rheumatology International*, **10**, 227–30.

Papers

Bastein, S. (1990). 'Patterns of neuropsychological abnormalities and cognitive impairment in adults and children'. Symposium on Myalgic Encephalomyelitis, Cambridge April 1990. Abstract, p. 6.

Bell, D. S., (1990). 'M.E./CFIDS in children: A historical overview'. Symposium on Myalgic Encephalomyelitis, Cambridge April 1990. Abstract, p. 6.

Doyle, D. (1990). 'Muscle biopsies in postviral fatigue syndrome'. Symposium on Myalgic Encephalomyelitis, Cambridge, April 1990. Abstract, p. 9.

Durndell, A. (1989). '2nd report to health and safety committee on postviral fatigue syndrome or myalgic encephalomyelitis', Glasgow College.

Goldstein, J. A. (1990). 'Presumed pathogenesis and treatment of the chronic fatigue syndrome/fibromyalgia complex'. Conference on Chronic Fatigue Syndrome and Fibromyalgia, Los Angeles, Feb. 1990. Abstract, p. 8.

Levine, S., Trestman, R., Halper, J., and Cunningham-Rundles, C. (1990). 'Plasma catecholamines in patients with chronic fatigue syndrome.' Abstract Presented at the American Psychiatric Association, May 1990.

Warner, C. L. (1990). 'Neuromuscular abnormalities in patients with M.E.'. Symposium on Myalgic Encephalomyelitis, Cambridge, April 1990. Abstract, p. 29.

List of Abbreviations

ACE	Advisory Centre for Education
ACTH	adrenocorticotrophic hormone
AIDS	acquired immune deficiency syndrome
ARMS	Action for Research into Multiple Sclerosis
CFIDS	chronic fatigue and immune dysfunction syndrome
CFS	chronic fatigue syndrome
CRH	corticotrophin releasing hormone
DNA	deoxyribonucleic acid
DSS	Department of Social Security
EB virus	Epstein Barr virus
ECG	electrocardiogram
EEG	electroencephalogram
EFAs	essential fatty acids
EMG	electromyography
EPA	eicosapentaenoeic acid
EPO	evening primrose oil
EPD	enzyme potentiated desensitization
GLA	gamma linolenic acid
HBLV	human B-cell lymphotropic virus
HBO	hyperbaric oxygen
HHV-6	human herpes virus type 6
IgA, IgG, IgM	immunoglobulin A (G,M)
MAOIs	monoamine oxidase inhibitors
ME	myalgic encephalomyelitis
MEAC	ME Action Campaign
MRI	magnetic resonance imaging
MS	multiple sclerosis

NHS	National Health Service
NI	National Insurance
NK cells	natural killer cells
NMR	nuclear magnetic resonance
PCR	polymerase chain reaction
PGE1	prostaglandin E 1
PMS	premenstrual syndrome
PMT	premenstrual tension
PVFS	postviral fatigue syndrome
RDA	recommended daily allowance
REM	rapid eye movement
RNA	ribonucleic acid
SLE	systemic lupus erythematosis
TM	transcendental meditation
VDUs	visual display units
VP1	virus protein 1

Index